SYPHILIS – RECOGNITION, DESCRIPTION AND DIAGNOSIS

Edited by **Neuza S. Sato**

Syphilis – Recognition, Description and Diagnosis
Edited by Neuza S. Sato

Published by InTech
Janeza Trdine 9, 51000 Rijeka, Croatia

Technical Editor Sonja Mujacic

Cover Designer InTech Design Team

Additional hard copies can be obtained from orders@intechopen.com

Syphilis – Recognition, Description and Diagnosis,
Edited by Edited by Neuza S. Sato
p. cm.
ISBN 978-953-307-554-9

For EU product safety concerns:
IN TECH d.o.o., Prolaz Marije Krucifikse Kozulić 3, 51000 Rijeka, Croatia,
info@intechopen.com or visit our website at intechopen.com.

Meet the editor

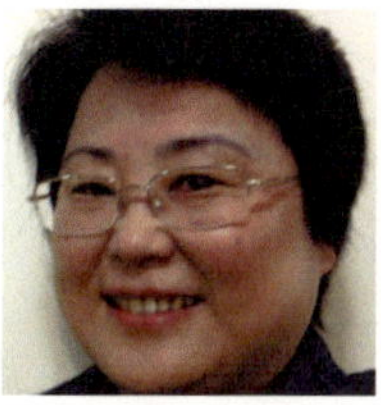

Dr. Neuza Satomi Sato is currently reseach fellow at Instituto Adolfo Lutz, a reference laboratory in Public Health situated in Sao Paulo city, Sao Paulo State, Brazil. She graduateed from the Faculty of Pharmaceutical Sciences from Universidade de São Paulo, and received a master and PhD degrees of Pharmacy from Universidade de Sao Paulo. She has experience in microbiology and biotechnology, acting in following subjects: research and development of new reagents and methods for laboratorial diagnosis and epidemiological studies of acquired and congenital infections. She is carrying out research related with syphilis disease since 1990.

Contents

Preface

Syphilis, a sexually transmitted disease was first described in 15th century. It is caused by *Treponema pallidum* subsp. *pallidum,* it occurs worldwide and it remains an important health problem.

This book collects chapters which present novel knowledge about the *T. pallidum,* some historical aspects of venereal disease and up to date information about syphilis disease.

First section includes chapters 1 and 2, which deal with novel knowledge of *T. pallidum:* The immunologic recognition of the etiologic agent of syphilis (*T. pallidum)* by the pattern recognition receptors of the innate immune system, and the identification of new targets for molecular diagnosis of *T.pallidum* by analysis of treponeme whole genome.

Second section includes chapters 3, 4 and 5, which present some information about Syphilis Disease: A historical aspects of venereal diseases treatment, a clinical aspects dealing with psychiatric manifestations of neurosyphilis and spatial and temporal patterns of primary syphilis and secondary syphilis described by the spatial and space-time scan statistics.

Finally, the last section includes chapters 6, 7 and 8, which mainly deal with laboratorial diagnosis of syphilis. A review of methods commonly used for laboratorial diagnosis, the serological response to treatment of syphilis and safety in blood transfusion.

I would like to thank each of the authors of the chapters, who took their great efforts in writing the articles, and sharing their knowledge, expertise and ideas for this book.

I wish to express my gratitude to Ms. Mirna Cvijic, InTech Publishing Process Manager, for her constant assistance and support during all phases of preparation of this book. I would also like to thank very much to Ms. Viktorija Zgela, editorial consultant at InTech, who contacted me to take over the editorial task of this project.

I am also indebted to InTech and its staff for the accomplishment of this book project.

Dr. Neuza Satomi Sato
Center of Immunology,
Institute Adolfo Lutz
São Paulo, SP
Brazil

Part 1

Treponema pallidum

1

Recognition of *Treponema pallidum* and Other Spirochetes by the Innate Immune System

Gunthard Stübs and Ralf R. Schumann
Charité – Universitätsmedizin Berlin, Berlin
Germany

1. Introduction

In 1905 the spirochete *T. pallidum* was discovered as the aetiologic agent of syphilis by Schaudinn and Hoffmann at the Charité Hospital in Berlin, Germany (Schaudinn & Hoffmann, 1905). This helical shaped bacterium is extremely well hidden, and also one of the best adapted to its only host – the Homo sapiens. The genome of *T. pallidum* ssp. *pallidum* contains only 1041 coding sequences and lacks numerous catabolic and biosynthetic pathways (Fraser et al., 1998) like, i.e. fatty acid synthesis (Livermore & Johnson, 1975). Therefore this organism utilises many of the biosynthetic precursors from its host and up to now it is not possible to continuously cultivate it *in vitro*. The only way to grow this bacterium is in *in vivo* models (Norris et al., 2006). Thus, the isolation of biological active compounds of *T. pallidum* has been difficult due to the lack of sufficient amounts of cultured bacteria. To study recognition of *T. pallidum* by the innate immune system information on the chemical composition of these cells has to be correlated with immunological responses induced by related spirochetes. The best examined spirochete is *Borrelia burgdorferi* – the etiologic agent of Lyme disease (LD). LD is an endemic disease with somewhat similar characteristics as compared to syphilis – A relatively slow dissemination of the spirochete within the host is followed by a weak inflammatory response of the human immune system. Furthermore, multiple organs are affected including the skin as well as the peripheral and central nervous system. Only half of the genes of *B. burgdorferi* code for proteins orthologous to those of *T. pallidum* indicating an adaptation to distinct niches though (Subramanian et al., 2000). However, the motility associated genes are highly conserved in both organisms (Fraser et al., 1998). Other pathogenic *Borrelia* include *B. hermsii*, one causative agent of relapsing fever, that multiplies more rapidly to higher cell numbers and causes more acute clinical symptoms. Further human associated treponemes such as *T. denticola*, colonise the oral cavity, *T. phagedenis*, belongs to the genital flora, and other species are found within the intestine. Thereof only the oral treponemes are pathogenic and have been associated with periodontal disease causing inflammation of the gingival tissue (Norris et al., 2006). Since the genome of *T. denticola* is much larger than that of *T. pallidum* and a conserved gene order could not be determined it is unlikely that *T. pallidum* is directly derived from this oral spirochete. But it might serve as a model for *T. pallidum* research since it is relatively easy to cultivate (Seshadri et al., 2004). While *Borrelia* and *Treponema* share the same phylogenetic family – *Spirochaetaceae* – the genus *Leptospira* belongs to the family *Leptospiraceae* in the same order as the first – *Spirochetales* (Paster et al., 1991). The most important and immunologically best studied leptospiral pathogen is the agent of Weil's disease (leptospirosis) *L. interrogans*.

1.1 The innate immune system

The innate immune system is the first line of defence of the host against invading microorganisms. Its function is to avoid an infection, or, in case an infection occurred, to detect, kill and eradicate the germs. Furthermore in vertebrates it interacts with the adaptive immune system and i.e. facilitates the presentation of antigens. The innate immune system mainly consists of either circulating or tissue resident cells, and humoral components like the complement system and cytokines. The phagocytes include the monocytes, macrophages, neutrophil granulocytes, or dendritic cells. These cells express germ-line encoded pattern recognition receptors (PRR) that detect conserved microbial structures not being present in the host. These receptor families include binding receptors like mannose binding receptors, CD14 or scavenger receptors like CD36. These proteins directly bind or mediate the binding of microbial patterns but they can't activate immune cells. The other PRRs are signalling receptors like toll-like (TLR), nod-like (NLR), or rig-I-like (RLR) receptors that usually contain a ligand-binding and a signalling domain. Upon ligand binding a conformational change within the signalling domain of the PRR triggers the signalling cascade inside the cell. This leads to the translocation of transcriptions factors into the nucleus and the release of cytokines (Akira & Takeda, 2004b).

1.2 The tools for receptor research

To assess the individual contribution of receptors of the innate immune response to a pathogen and the specificity of the ligands, loss-of-function and gain-of-function assays are used. There are mainly three ways to selectively disable single receptors in loss-of-function experiments. The most widely used system are knockout (KO) mice, in which receptor genes were turned off by homologous recombination in embryonic stem cells (Hemmi et al., 2000). Today numerous inbred KO mice are available either commercially or through research collaborations lacking relevant receptors or proteins of the signalling cascade (Akira & Takeda, 2004a). These animal models, however, do not always reflect the situation in humans. Genotyping of healthy volunteers for natural occurring functionally relevant mutations in the receptor genes allows experiments with isolated peripheral blood mononuclear cells from humans. Finally, loss-of-function experiments can be designed by downregulation of genes by small interfering RNA (siRNA) (Elbashir et al., 2001). Upon transfection of these plasmids into cells they interfere with the translation of the targeted mRNA leading to degradation of the mRNA prior to translation and a strong reduction of the receptor protein expression (knockdown). The most widely used assay for gain-of-function experiments are cell lines like the human embryonic kidney cells (HEK 293). In these epithelial cells numerous PRRs are either not expressed or expressed only dysfunctional while the signalling cascade is mostly intact. By transfection of receptor plasmids it is possible to study cellular activation upon stimulation with bacterial ligands in contrast to non-transfected cells. The read-out for these experiments are either cytokines like IL-8 or reporter-gene assays for transcription factors like NF-κB (Opitz et al., 2001). If working with novel isolated bacterial structures it is useful to first check their biological activity with cell lines that express a full set of PRRs. The most often used cell lines are human monocytes like THP-1 or the murine macrophages RAW 264.7 (Schröder et al., 2000).

1.3 The morphology and the cell wall composition of *T. pallidum*

Spirochetes stain negative in Gram-staining and share the main cell wall topology of Gram-negative bacteria. In detail the *T. pallidum* envelope is assembled by an outer and a cytoplasmic (inner) membrane enclosing the protoplasmic cylinder (Johnson et al., 1973).

The periplasmic space is constituted by a thin peptidoglycan layer (Umemoto et al., 1981) and anchors the endoflagella (also called axial filaments) (Johnson et al., 1973). From the centre of the cell the endoflagella wrap around the protoplasmic cylinder and extend at each end into the extracellular space (Hovind-Hougen, 1976). The outer membrane contains few transmembrane proteins (Jones et al., 1995; Radolf et al., 1989; Walker et al., 1989) and exhibits an extremely low protein/lipid ratio (Radolf, Robinson, Bourell, Akins, Porcella, Weigel, Jones & Norgard, 1995). Hydrophobic proteins are anchored in both membranes (Radolf et al., 1988). The majority, however, is located in the cytoplasmic membrane (Cox et al., 1995). Both membranes themselves are mainly constituted of lipids that comprise about 20 % of the dry weight of *T. pallidum* cells (Johnson et al., 1970). About 50 % of the total lipids are attributed to the glycolipid α-galactosyl-diacylglycerol (MGalD) (Livermore & Johnson, 1970) while about 45 % are phosphatidylcholine and -ethanolamine, which are found in the host too. The remaining portion are free fatty acids (Johnson et al., 1970). With more sensitive radiolabelling assays further phospholipids have been detected in minor proportions (Belisle et al., 1994). The peptidoglycan layer consists chemically of an oligomer of glucosamine and muramic acid that is cross linked by short peptides (Umemoto et al., 1981).

2. Toll-like receptors

Toll-like receptors (TLR) are single-pass transmembrane receptors. Within the cell one group is located on the cellular surface, the other within endosomes. They exhibit an ecto-domain containing leucine-rich repeats detecting the ligands, a transmembrane domain, and a cytoplasmic domain inducing signal transduction. This intracellular domain is termed toll/IL-1R (TIR) domain due to its homology to the IL-1 receptor signalling domain (Fig. 1, p. 4). Adaptor molecules associated with the TIR domain trigger intracellular signalling, with MyD88 being the central signal transducer (Akira & Takeda, 2004a). TLRs are not only expressed in cells of the innate immune system but partially in B lymphocytes and endothelial cells too. They are named according to their homology with the toll protein found in *Drosophila*. In 1997 the first human TLR was cloned and its function for the signalling of the immune system discovered (Medzhitov et al., 1997). Subsequently a protein family consisting of 10 members in humans was identified and numerous ligands proposed. Prior to these findings immunstimulatory molecules such as lipoproteins from *T. pallidum* (Norgard et al., 1995) or lipopolysaccharide from Gram-negative bacteria as well as the involvement of some binding receptors were established but the signalling receptor and the entire mechanism remained unknown.

2.1 TLR-4

TLR-4 is responsible for the recognition of lipopolysaccharides (LPS) (Poltorak et al., 1998; Qureshi et al., 1999) but binding assays revealed that MD-2, an accessory protein of TLR-4 receptor complex, directly binds LPS. Due to the association of MD-2 with a homodimer of TLR-4 it triggers signalling (Shimazu et al., 1999; Viriyakosol et al., 2000). Earlier it was found that the serum protein LPS binding protein (LBP) (Schumann et al., 1990) and membrane bound or soluble CD14 (Wright et al., 1990) are also involved in the recognition cascade of LPS. Both facilitate recognition of LPS by TLR-4 in the pg/ml range. All these membrane bound proteins are localised on the cell surface. LPS is an amphiphilic molecule that is located in the outer leaflet of the outer membrane of Gram-negative bacteria. Chemically it is composed of lipid A, a phosphorylated disaccharide with 4-6 attached fatty acids including hydroxy fatty acids, and the core region, an oligosaccharide with the characteristic carbohydrate

3-deoxy-D-manno-octulosonic acid (KDO). The active principle for binding to MD-2 and initiating signalling is lipid A (Viriyakosol et al., 2000).

Spirochetes share the cell wall design of Gram-negative bacteria but they seem to lack a classical TLR-4 stimulating LPS. This has been shown for *T. pallidum* (Hardy & Levin, 1983; Penn et al., 1985; Radolf & Norgard, 1988) as well as several *Borrelia* including *B. burgdorferi* (Hardy & Levin, 1983; Takayama et al., 1987). For *L. interrogans* an atypical LPS was reported (Vinh et al., 1986) and the chemical structure identified (Que-Gewirth et al., 2004). But this LPS is atypically recognised by TLR-2 instead of TLR-4 (Werts et al., 2001). In contrast several authors have reported on the putative isolation of LPS in *Treponema* (Kurimoto et al., 1990; Walker et al., 1999) and in *Borrelia* (Beck et al., 1985; Habicht et al., 1986). However, these findings are not convincing since the extracts are crude and not purified chemically. Furthermore, not all features of an LPS were found, and no chemical structure has been determined. Most importantly no activation of TLR-4 has been reported. Therefore it appears obvious that TLR-4 is not relevant in recognition of *T. pallidum* and spirochetes in general.

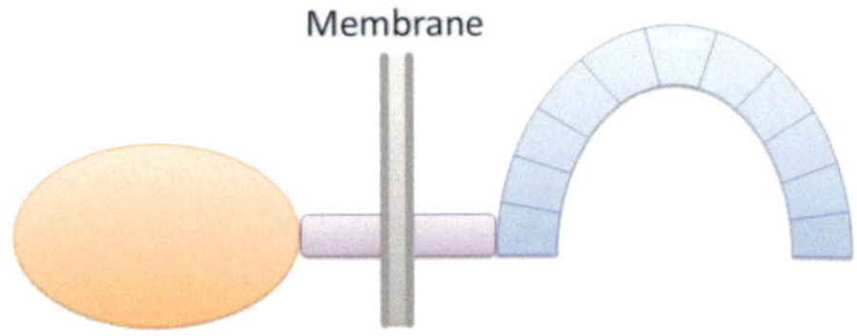

Fig. 1. Schematic representation of the basic structure of toll-like receptors

2.2 TLR-2, TLR-1, TLR-6

The first ligands described for TLR-2 were bacterial lipoproteins (Aliprantis et al., 1999; Brightbill et al., 1999; Lien et al., 1999). Later it has been shown that TLR-2 forms heterodimers with either TLR-1 or TLR-6 to recognise triacylated and diacylated lipoproteins, respectively (Takeuchi et al., 2001; 2002), and the crystal structures of both ligands in complex with the respective receptor dimer have been elucidated (Jin et al., 2007; Kang et al., 2009). For signalling via the TLR-1/-6 receptor complex CD36 is a crucial cofactor (Hoebe et al., 2005). TLR-1, -2 and -6 are located on the cellular surface as well (Kawai & Akira, 2009). Further ligands of diverse chemical nature have been proposed for TLR-2 and today it is the TLR with the highest number of proposed ligands. However, since the biological activity of bacterial lipoproteins and peptides in the upper pg/ml range (Schröder et al., 2004) is highest among the TLR-2 ligands, lipoproteins can be considered as the prototype TLR-2-ligand. The biological importance of bacterial lipoproteins is to anchor proteins into cellular membranes. Its chemical structure was first described in 1973 (Hantke & Braun, 1973). The basic structure of the lipid anchor is a diacylglycerol molecule that is thioether linked to a cysteine. The cysteine constitutes the N-terminal amino acid of the protein. In case of triacylated lipoproteins the N-terminal amino group is amide linked to a further fatty acid. The biosynthetic pathway is ubiquitous in bacteria and lipoproteins have been predicted in many bacteria (Madan Babu & Sankaran, 2002). The active principle for the recognition by TLR-2 heterodimers is the lipid anchor and not the protein moiety.

2.2.1 Bacterial lipoproteins in *T. pallidum*

Due to the complete genome sequencing and known signalling peptides numerous putative lipoproteins could be predicted in the microbes sequenced: 46 in *T. pallidum* (22 by Fraser et al. (1998)), 166 in *T. denticola* and 127 in *B. burgdorferi* according to new algorithms (Setubal et al., 2006). For *B. burgdorferi* it has been shown previously that their lipoproteins are triacylated (Beermann et al., 2000). Since in *T. pallidum* the necessary enzyme for the acylation of the N-terminus – apolipoprotein N-acyltransferase – is present[1], it is likely that its lipoproteins are triacylated as well. A fraction of lipoproteins from *T. pallidum* has been isolated (Chamberlain et al., 1989; Radolf et al., 1988) and shown to activate isolated murine macrophages and the cell line RAW 264.7 (Radolf et al., 1991). These results could be confirmed by the biological activity of fully synthetic lipopeptides (DeOgny et al., 1994) that are able to mimic inflammation *in vivo* (Norgard et al., 1995). This activity has been shown to employ a distinct receptor then LPS (Norgard et al., 1996) but involves CD14 (Sellati et al., 1998) and LBP (Schröder et al., 2004). Furthermore it has been demonstrated that the acylation of the lipid anchor is an essential feature for recognition (Morr et al., 2002; Radolf et al., 1995). The lipoproteins of *T. pallidum* and *B. burgdorferi* and their lipopeptide analogs have been used as a model to identify TLR-2 as the signalling receptor (Lien et al., 1999). However the heterodimer partner for *T. pallidum* lipoproteins remains undetermined. For oral treponemes the recognition of bacteria or cell wall components by TLR-2 has been reported (Asai et al., 2003). In case of *T. denticola* the heterodimer TLR-2/-6 is utilised for signalling indicating rather a diacylated lipoprotein (Ruby et al., 2007). Since lipoproteins of *T. denticola* have been described as activating murine macrophages prior to the knowledge of TLR-2 (Rosen et al., 1999) it is likely that they exhibit the same TLR-2 activity as *T. pallidum*. Probably lipoproteins are the most important TLR ligands of *T. pallidum* and spirochetes in general. In *B. hermsii* TLR-2 is crucial for the activation of the adaptive immune system and production of antibodies (Dickinson et al., 2010).

2.2.2 Glycostructures in treponemes

Polysaccharides have been isolated from treponemes and subjected to compositional analyses indicating many kinds of carbohydrates (Yanagihara et al., 1984). Amphiphilic glycostructures from the outer membrane of *T. denticola* were isolated but no defined chemical structure was elucidated (Schultz et al., 1998). Similar not further chemically purified glycostructures were obtained from culture supernatants of *T. maltophilum*, an oral treponeme, or extracted from the same cells. These have been shown to activate murine macrophages as well as cell lines in a TLR-2-dependent fashion but only in very high concentrations (μg/ml) (Opitz et al., 2001; Schröder et al., 2000). However contaminations with lipoproteins that have similar hydrophobic properties like these amphiphilic glycostructures could not be ruled out.

2.3 TLR-5

TLR-5 detects bacterial flagellin of several Gram-positive and Gram-negative bacteria. The receptor binds this protein directly and leads to NF-κB activation and release of proinflammatory cytokines (Hayashi et al., 2001; Smith et al., 2003). The recognised monomeric FlaA is highly conserved and a principle component of the flagellar filaments. It is essential for the motility of bacteria. Unlike other TLRs, TLR-5 is not expressed on macrophages or dendritic cells but mainly on intestinal cells (Uematsu et al., 2006). *T. pallidum* features several endoflagella that consist of flagellin too. The genetic analyses of the flagellar structure reveal that *T. pallidum* has three core proteins (FlaB1-3) and one sheath protein (FlaA) while in *B. burgdorferi* a single core and one sheath protein is found (Fraser et al., 1998). Of the

[1] http://www.ncbi.nlm.nih.gov/gene/6333053

spirochetes only for *B. burgdorferi* the role of TLR-5 has been assessed: Upon stimulation with live bacteria knockdown of the TLR-5 gene by siRNA resulted in either a minor effect (Dennis et al., 2009) or a significant reduction of cytokine gene expression (Shin et al., 2008). A direct stimulation of cells with the FlaA gene product (p37) increased the protein level of TLR-5 (Cabral et al., 2006). Taken the presence of FlaA in *T. pallidum* , its high conservation among bacteria, and the first results on the TLR-5 role in *B. burgdorferi*, TLR-5 probably contributes to the recognition of *T. pallidum* too. However, this fact and the extent of the signalling remains to be elucidated.

2.4 TLR-9

TLR-9 was identified as the PRR for unmethylated 2′-deoxyribo cytidine-phosphate-guanosine (CpG) DNA motifs (Hemmi et al., 2000). The general immune stimulatory effects of these motifs were already established prior to the discovery of TLR-9. In contrast to mammals in bacteria CpG DNA motifs are 20 times more common (Klinman et al., 1996). First it was assumed that the recognition is species specific via the nucleotide sequence of the CpG motifs (Bauer et al., 2001) while it was later revealed that the DNA carbohydrate backbone 2′ deoxyribose determines the activation of TLR-9 (Haas et al., 2008). This receptor is expressed in intracellular vesicles like endosomes. No results on the role of TLR-9 in the immune response to *T. pallidum* have been reported. For *B. burgdorferi* the production of proinflammatory cytokines in TLR-9 deficient murine macrophages was not diminished compared to wild-type macrophages (Shin et al., 2008). In contrast, the interferon α production induced by *B. burgdorferi* was significantly reduced upon TLR-9 inhibition (Petzke et al., 2009) and *B. hermsii* activates TLR-9 (Dickinson et al., 2010). However it remains an open issue whether also the DNA of *T. pallidum* could be recognised by TLR-9.

TLRs -3, -7, and -8 are located in intracellular compartments. They sense double (-3) and single stranded (-7, -8) RNA found in RNA viruses. Therefore these TLRs don't appear to be relevant for the innate immune recognition of spirochetes. For the human TLR-10 currently no clear ligand is known (Kawai & Akira, 2009).

3. Nod-like receptors

Nucleotide oligomerisation domain (NOD)-like receptors (NLRs) are a family of intracellular PRRs with 23 members in humans. They are expressed in many cell types but some primarily in phagocytes. The NLRs are multi-domain proteins consisting of a nucleotide-binding domain, leucine-rich repeats (LRR) and an N-terminal effector domain (Fig. 2). Similar to the TLRs the LRR bind the microbial structures while the effector domain triggers the signalling cascade leading to activation of mitogen-activated protein (MAP) kinase, translocation of NF-κB, or activation of the inflammasome (Franchi et al., 2009). The best characterised NLRs are NOD-1 and NOD-2 that sense substructures of the bacterial peptidoglycan (PG) (Ting et al., 2008).

3.1 NOD-2

NOD-2 has been revealed as the receptor for muramyldipeptide (MDP) from Gram-positive and Gram-negative bacteria. Upon binding of the ligand it triggers the activation of NF-κB pathway (Girardin et al., 2003b; Inohara et al., 2003). The immunstimulatory properties of MDP were known a long time before and it has been widely used as an adjuvant (in Freund's complete adjuvant) (Chedid, 1983). Furthermore it has been shown that MDP synergises with LPS in the induction of proinflammatory cytokine release (Takada et al., 2002; Wang et al., 2001). NOD-2 is predominantly expressed in the cytosol of monocytes/macrophages (Girardin et al., 2003b). Chemically MDP is N-acetylmuramyl-L-alanyl-D-isoglutamine and it is the minimal glycosubstructure of PG also from spirochetes. For *T. pallidum* the basic MDP components muramic acid, alanine and glutamic acid[2] have been detected in its PG (Azuma et al., 1975). However the exact sequence of the glycan linking peptides and therefore the structural requirement for NOD-2 recognition in treponemes is still unknown. In one report the treponemal PG lacked the adjuvant activity to stimulate antibody production (Umemoto et al., 1981). Early reports on the biological activity of PG from *B. burgdorferi* (Beck et al., 1990) and from *T. denticola* (Grenier & Uitto, 1993) can't be included since the PG preparations were not devoid of lipoproteins and no specific receptors were assessed. Nevertheless for LD an important role of NOD-2 in an interplay with TLR-2 was demonstrated recently. Both receptors are necessary for an effective induction of cytokines by *B. burgdorferi* (Oosting et al., 2010). Also *B. hermsii* activates NOD-2 (Dickinson et al., 2010). Since *Borrelia* and *Treponema* are supposed to have the same PG composition the role of NOD-2 in the recognition of the syphilis spirochete should be examined.

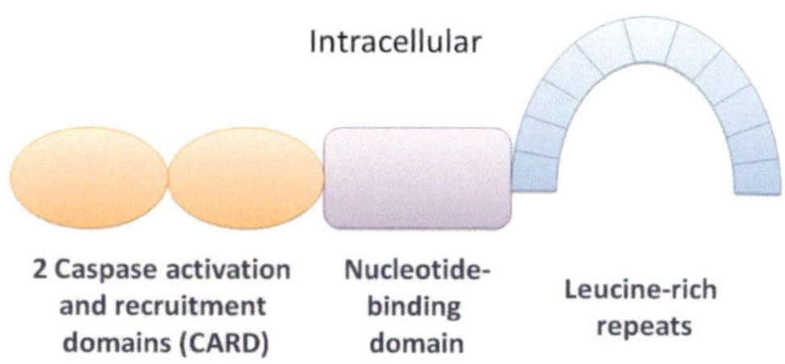

Fig. 2. Schematic representation of the structure of NOD-2 receptor

3.2 NOD-1

NOD-1 is the sensing PRR for another PG motif, the iE-DAP dipeptide of the glycan strand cross linking peptide (Chamaillard et al., 2003; Girardin et al., 2003a). The receptor-ligand complex then leads to the activation of NF-κB and cytokine release as well. NOD-1 is expressed in the cytosol of multiple tissues (Chamaillard et al., 2003). The unique part of the ligand iE-DAP (γ-D-glutamyl-*meso*-diaminopimelic acid) is the diaminopimelic acid. In general all common Gram-negative and only several Gram-positive bacteria exhibit this diamino acid. In spirochetes it was only detected in *Leptospira* while in contrast *Treponema* and *Borrelia* contain the diamino acid ornithine instead (Umemoto et al., 1981; Yanagihara et al., 1984). Furthermore, for *B. burgdorferi* it has been shown that NOD-1 plays no major role in the recognition by the immune system (Oosting et al., 2010) and the same is expected for *T. pallidum*.

4. CD1d

CD1d is a surface glycoprotein similar to the MHC class I molecules that presents lipid antigens to invariant natural killer T cells (iNKT). The iNKT cells are a small subset of T lymphocytes that express an invariant $\alpha\beta$ T cell receptor as well as a NK cell receptor. They activate monocytes and B-cells by immunregulatory cytokines linking the innate and adaptive immune system (Cohen et al., 2009). This seems to be an important mechanism for production of antilipid antibodies too (Leadbetter et al., 2008). For LD it has been shown

[2] during the applied compositional analysis isoglutamine will be converted to glutamic acid

that CD1d deficiency impairs the host resistance to *B. burgdorferi* in a mouse model (Kumar et al., 2000). In line with this is the observation that iNKT deficient mice exhibit more severe and prolonged manifestations as well as a reduced ability to clear the spirochetes (Tupin et al., 2008). This effect could be attributed to one of the *B. burgdorferi* glycolipids namely α-galactosyl-diacylglycerol (MGalD) (Fig. 3b) that activates iNKT cells via CD1d and independent of TLRs (Kinjo et al., 2006). MGalD is structurally related to the prototype iNKT cell ligand α-galactosylceramide (Fig. 3a) and shows the essential α-configuration of the galactose (Kawano et al., 1997). Furthermore for tick-borne relapsing fever it was demonstrated that CD1d deficiency coincides with impaired antibody production and increased *B. hermsii* burden (Belperron et al., 2005). Due to the fact that *B. hermsii* lipids contain MGalD too (Livermore et al., 1978) a crucial role of CD1d and its ligand MGalD in the defence of *Borrelia* can be concluded. For syphilis the role of CD1d and iNKT cells have not been assessed so far. However while in *B. hermsii* and *B. burgdorferi* MGalD comprises for 2.6 % and 3.4 % of cell dry weight respectively (Stübs et al., 2009) in *T. pallidum* MGalD is the major lipid structure accounting for 9-10 % of the dry bacterial cell (Johnson et al., 1970; Livermore & Johnson, 1970). Therefore we hypothesize that for syphilis the activation of iNKT cells by CD1d and treponemal MGalD is an important mechanism for the innate as well as the adaptive immune response.

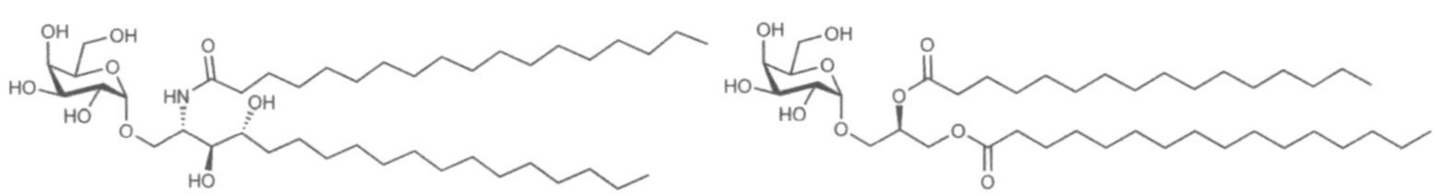

(a) α-Galactosylceramide (b) α-Galactosyl-diacylglycerol

Fig. 3. Chemical structures of CD1d ligands

5. Phagocytosis

In vivo the host's immune cells are faced first with live bacteria which do not expose the epitops for the PRRs to the surface. For *B. hermsii* the crucial role of the initial bacterial cell degradation has been demonstrated: Blocking of internalisation of the bacterial cell prevents the induction of inflammatory cytokines (Dickinson et al., 2010). Hence, prior to TLR/NLR recognition and signalling an effective phagocytosis of bacteria is important. At first the phagocytes have to rely on their low affinity binding receptors and the complement opsonins to attach the bacteria. In a later stage of the immune response highly specific IgG antibodies can opsonise the bacteria and allow the phagocytes to bind their F_C moiety with much higher affinity. Thereafter immune cells ingest and lyse the bacteria in the phagolysosome. For live *T. pallidum* the phagocytosis proceeds considerably slower than with other bacteria (Alder et al., 1990). Compared to *B. burgdorferi* it results in significantly weaker activation of monocytes and less release of cytokines. Only in the presence of syphilic sera *T. pallidum* initiates an equally efficient immune response as compared to *B. burgdorferi* (Moore et al., 2007). For the uptake of *B. burgdorferi* the adaptor molecule MyD88 but not TLR-2, -5 and -9 is important and plays a dual role – for signal transduction and for phagocytosis (Shin et al., 2008). Breaking down the bacterial polymers to small subunits is not only obvious for the mentioned NLRs but also for TLR-5. Here the acidic environment in the phagolysosome is necessary to disperse the filament into the monomeric flagellin (Smith et al., 2003).

6. Conclusion

The first crucial step for immune responses upon infection with *T. pallidum* is its degradation in order to have the ligands available for PRRs of the innate immune system. However, during early syphilis IgG antibodies are absent and phagocytosis of *T. pallidum* is markedly weak. Therefore only limited amounts of treponemal ligands are recognised by PRRs rendering low inflammation. Furthermore pyrogenicity of *T. pallidum*, lacking the highly active LPS, is diminished in regard to Gram-negative bacteria. The most potent PRR ligands in *T. pallidum* are lipoproteins recognised by TLR-2. Compared to *B. burgdorferi* the number of distinct lipoproteins is more limited but no conclusion as to the overall expression can be drawn. Since the activation of the innate immune system by *T. pallidum* and *B. burgdorferi* is similar in extent, it appears that TLR-5, recognizing flagellin, and TLR-9, recognizing DNA, play a role for recognition of *T. pallidum* as well. Both ligands are present in *T. pallidum* from the genetic and chemical point of view but remaining uncertainty has to be assessed by experiments with treponemal ligands. The same holds true for the activation of immune cells by MDP via NOD-2. Chemical analyses indicate the presence of the MDP motif but further evidence has to be gathered. The role of TLR-1 and -6 as heterodimers of TLR-2 have not been elucidated finally. However, the presence of triacylated lipoproteins in *T. pallidum* rather suggests a function of TLR-1. The other TLRs and NOD-1 are probably not involved in *T. pallidum* recognition. The presentation of treponemal MGalD by CD1d to iNKT cells is a novel aspect presented here first and should be studied in detail.

Thus, the weak phagocytosis combined with the reduced recognition of *T. pallidum* by the PRRs can explain its "stealth" during the first stages of syphilis. In the absence of IgG antibodies *T. pallidum* induces only weak inflammation and leads to painless ulcerations as in the primary stage. Insufficient recognition and eradication enables *T. pallidum* to disseminate by the blood stream and lymphatic system and affect other organs as in the second stage of syphilis. Furthermore the weak activation of the innate immune system results in diminished presentation of antigens for adaptive immune responses. The following delayed production of IgM and more pronounced IgG antibodies has been observed by serodiagnostics. However, in late stage syphilis IgG antibodies are present and an efficient phagocytosis has been demonstrated *in vitro*. At this time *T. pallidum* can only persist in the host due to evasion into organs with restricted immune responses as the central nervous system. In late syphilis dissemination of *T. pallidum* within the host is prevented and the host is not infectious anymore.

Taken together different characteristics of *T. pallidum* allow it to evade the immune response of the host – passively to disseminate during early syphilis and actively to establish a chronic infection. For both features the interaction with the innate immune system is pivotal.

7. References

Akira, S. & Takeda, K. (2004a). Functions of toll-like receptors: lessons from ko mice, *C R Biol* 327(6): 581–9.

Akira, S. & Takeda, K. (2004b). Toll-like receptor signalling, *Nat Rev Immunol* 4(7): 499–511.

Alder, J. D., Friess, L., Tengowski, M. & Schell, R. F. (1990). Phagocytosis of opsonized treponema pallidum subsp. pallidum proceeds slowly, *Infect Immun* 58(5): 1167–73.

Aliprantis, A. O., Yang, R. B., Mark, M. R., Suggett, S., Devaux, B., Radolf, J. D., Klimpel, G. R., Godowski, P. & Zychlinsky, A. (1999). Cell activation and apoptosis by bacterial lipoproteins through toll-like receptor-2, *Science* 285(5428): 736–9.

Asai, Y., Jinno, T. & Ogawa, T. (2003). Oral treponemes and their outer membrane extracts activate human gingival epithelial cells through toll-like receptor 2, *Infect. Immun.* 71(2): 717–25.

Azuma, I., Taniyama, T., Yamamura, Y., Yanagihara, Y. & Hattori, Y. (1975). Chemical studies on the cell walls of leptorspira biflexa strain urawa and treponema pallidum strain reiter, *Jpn J Microbiol* 19(1): 45–51.

Bauer, S., Kirschning, C. J., Hacker, H., Redecke, V., Hausmann, S., Akira, S., Wagner, H. & Lipford, G. B. (2001). Human tlr9 confers responsiveness to bacterial dna via species-specific cpg motif recognition, *Proc. Natl. Acad. Sci. USA* 98(16): 9237–42.

Beck, G., Benach, J. L. & Habicht, G. S. (1990). Isolation, preliminary chemical characterization, and biological activity of borrelia burgdorferi peptidoglycan, *Biochem. Biophys. Res. Commun.* 167(1): 89–95.

Beck, G., Habicht, G. S., Benach, J. L. & Coleman, J. L. (1985). Chemical and biologic characterization of a lipopolysaccharide extracted from the lyme disease spirochete (borrelia burgdorferi), *J. Infect. Dis.* 152(1): 108–17.

Beermann, C., Lochnit, G., Geyer, R., Groscurth, P. & Filgueira, L. (2000). The lipid component of lipoproteins from borrelia burgdorferi: structural analysis, antigenicity, and presentation via human dendritic cells, *Biochem. Biophys. Res. Commun.* 267(3): 897–905.

Belisle, J. T., Brandt, M. E., Radolf, J. D. & Norgard, M. V. (1994). Fatty acids of treponema pallidum and borrelia burgdorferi lipoproteins, *J. Bacteriol.* 176(8): 2151–7.

Belperron, A. A., Dailey, C. M. & Bockenstedt, L. K. (2005). Infection-induced marginal zone b cell production of borrelia hermsii-specific antibody is impaired in the absence of cd1d, *J Immunol* 174(9): 5681–6.

Brightbill, H. D., Libraty, D. H., Krutzik, S. R., Yang, R. B., Belisle, J. T., Bleharski, J. R., Maitland, M., Norgard, M. V., Plevy, S. E., Smale, S. T., Brennan, P. J., Bloom, B. R., Godowski, P. J. & Modlin, R. L. (1999). Host defense mechanisms triggered by microbial lipoproteins through toll-like receptors, *Science* 285(5428): 732–6.

Cabral, E. S., Gelderblom, H., Hornung, R. L., Munson, P. J., Martin, R. & Marques, A. R. (2006). Borrelia burgdorferi lipoprotein-mediated tlr2 stimulation causes the down-regulation of tlr5 in human monocytes, *J Infect Dis* 193(6): 849–59.

Chamaillard, M., Hashimoto, M., Horie, Y., Masumoto, J., Qiu, S., Saab, L., Ogura, Y., Kawasaki, A., Fukase, K., Kusumoto, S., Valvano, M. A., Foster, S. J., Mak, T. W., Nunez, G. & Inohara, N. (2003). An essential role for nod1 in host recognition of bacterial peptidoglycan containing diaminopimelic acid, *Nat. Immunol.* 4(7): 702–7.

Chamberlain, N. R., Brandt, M. E., Erwin, A. L., Radolf, J. D. & Norgard, M. V. (1989). Major integral membrane protein immunogens of treponema pallidum are proteolipids, *Infect. Immun.* 57(9): 2872–7.

Chedid, L. (1983). Muramyl peptides as possible endogenous immunopharmacological mediators, *Microbiol Immunol* 27(9): 723–32.

Cohen, N. R., Garg, S. & Brenner, M. B. (2009). Antigen presentation by cd1 lipids, t cells, and nkt cells in microbial immunity, *Adv Immunol* 102: 1–94.

Cox, D. L., Akins, D. R., Porcella, S. F., Norgard, M. V. & Radolf, J. D. (1995). Treponema pallidum in gel microdroplets: a novel strategy for investigation of treponemal molecular architecture, *Mol Microbiol* 15(6): 1151–64.

Dennis, V. A., Dixit, S., O'Brien, S. M., Alvarez, X., Pahar, B. & Philipp, M. T. (2009). Live borrelia burgdorferi spirochetes elicit inflammatory mediators from human monocytes via the toll-like receptor signaling pathway, *Infect Immun* 77(3): 1238–45.

DeOgny, L., Pramanik, B. C., Arndt, L. L., Jones, J. D., Rush, J., Slaughter, C. A., Radolf, J. D. & Norgard, M. V. (1994). Solid-phase synthesis of biologically active lipopeptides as analogs for spirochetal lipoproteins, *Pept. Res.* 7(2): 91–7.

Dickinson, G. S., Piccone, H., Sun, G., Lien, E., Gatto, L. & Alugupalli, K. R. (2010). Toll-like receptor 2 deficiency results in impaired antibody responses and septic shock during borrelia hermsii infection, *Infect Immun* 78(11): 4579–88.

Elbashir, S. M., Harborth, J., Lendeckel, W., Yalcin, A., Weber, K. & Tuschl, T. (2001). Duplexes of 21-nucleotide rnas mediate rna interference in cultured mammalian cells, *Nature* 411(6836): 494–8.

Franchi, L., Warner, N., Viani, K. & Nunez, G. (2009). Function of nod-like receptors in microbial recognition and host defense, *Immunol. Rev.* 227(1): 106–28.

Fraser, C. M., Norris, S. J., Weinstock, G. M., White, O., Sutton, G. G., Dodson, R., Gwinn, M., Hickey, E. K., Clayton, R., Ketchum, K. A., Sodergren, E., Hardham, J. M., McLeod, M. P., Salzberg, S., Peterson, J., Khalak, H., Richardson, D., Howell, J. K., Chidambaram, M., Utterback, T., McDonald, L., Artiach, P., Bowman, C., Cotton, M. D., Venter, J. C. & et al. (1998). Complete genome sequence of treponema pallidum, the syphilis spirochete, *Science* 281(5375): 375–88.

Girardin, S. E., Boneca, I. G., Carneiro, L. A., Antignac, A., Jehanno, M., Viala, J., Tedin, K., Taha, M. K., Labigne, A., Zähringer, U., Coyle, A. J., DiStefano, P. S., Bertin, J., Sansonetti, P. J. & Philpott, D. J. (2003). Nod1 detects a unique muropeptide from gram-negative bacterial peptidoglycan, *Science* 300(5625): 1584–7.

Girardin, S. E., Boneca, I. G., Viala, J., Chamaillard, M., Labigne, A., Thomas, G., Philpott, D. J. & Sansonetti, P. J. (2003). Nod2 is a general sensor of peptidoglycan through muramyl dipeptide (mdp) detection, *J. Biol. Chem.* 278(11): 8869–72.

Grenier, D. & Uitto, V. J. (1993). Cytotoxic effect of peptidoglycan from treponema denticola, *Microb Pathog* 15(5): 389–97.

Haas, T., Metzger, J., Schmitz, F., Heit, A., MALller, T., Latz, E. & Wagner, H. (2008). The dna sugar backbone 2′ deoxyribose determines toll-like receptor 9 activation, *Immunity* 28(3): 315–23.

Habicht, G. S., Beck, G., Benach, J. L. & Coleman, J. L. (1986). Borrelia burgdorferi lipopolysaccharide and its role in the pathogenesis of lyme disease, *Zentralbl. Bakteriol. Mikrobiol. Hyg. [A]* 263(1-2): 137–41.

Hantke, K. & Braun, V. (1973). Covalent binding of lipid to protein. diglyceride and amide-linked fatty acid at the n-terminal end of the murein-lipoprotein of the escherichia coli outer membrane, *Eur. J. Biochem.* 34(2): 284–96.

Hardy, P. H., J. & Levin, J. (1983). Lack of endotoxin in borrelia hispanica and treponema pallidum, *Proc. Soc. Exp. Biol. Med.* 174(1): 47–52.

Hayashi, F., Smith, K. D., Ozinsky, A., Hawn, T. R., Yi, E. C., Goodlett, D. R., Eng, J. K., Akira, S., Underhill, D. M. & Aderem, A. (2001). The innate immune response to bacterial flagellin is mediated by toll-like receptor 5, *Nature* 410(6832): 1099–103.

Hemmi, H., Takeuchi, O., Kawai, T., Kaisho, T., Sato, S., Sanjo, H., Matsumoto, M., Hoshino, K., Wagner, H., Takeda, K. & Akira, S. (2000). A toll-like receptor recognizes bacterial dna, *Nature* 408(6813): 740–5.

Hoebe, K., Georgel, P., Rutschmann, S., Du, X., Mudd, S., Crozat, K., Sovath, S., Shamel, L., Hartung, T., Zähringer, U. & Beutler, B. (2005). Cd36 is a sensor of diacylglycerides, *Nature* 433(7025): 523–7.

Hovind-Hougen, K. (1976). Determination by means of electron microscopy of morphological criteria of value for classification of some spirochetes, in particular treponemes, *Acta Pathol Microbiol Scand Suppl* (255): 1–41.

Inohara, N., Ogura, Y., Fontalba, A., Gutierrez, O., Pons, F., Crespo, J., Fukase, K., Inamura, S., Kusumoto, S., Hashimoto, M., Foster, S. J., Moran, A. P., Fernandez-Luna, J. L. & Nunez, G. (2003). Host recognition of bacterial muramyl dipeptide mediated through nod2. implications for crohn's disease, *J Biol Chem* 278(8): 5509–12.

Jin, M. S., Kim, S. E., Heo, J. Y., Lee, M. E., Kim, H. M., Paik, S. G., Lee, H. & Lee, J. O. (2007). Crystal structure of the tlr1-tlr2 heterodimer induced by binding of a tri-acylated lipopeptide, *Cell* 130(6): 1071–82.

Johnson, R. C., Livermore, B. P., Jenkin, H. M. & Eggebraten, L. (1970). Lipids of treponema pallidum kazan 5, *Infect. Immun.* 2(5): 606–609.

Johnson, R. C., Ritzi, D. M. & Livermore, B. P. (1973). Outer envelope of virulent treponema pallidum, *Infect. Immun.* 8(2): 291–5.

Jones, J. D., Bourell, K. W., Norgard, M. V. & Radolf, J. D. (1995). Membrane topology of borrelia burgdorferi and treponema pallidum lipoproteins, *Infect. Immun.* 63(7): 2424–34.

Kang, J. Y., Nan, X., Jin, M. S., Youn, S. J., Ryu, Y. H., Mah, S., Han, S. H., Lee, H., Paik, S. G. & Lee, J. O. (2009). Recognition of lipopeptide patterns by toll-like receptor 2-toll-like receptor 6 heterodimer, *Immunity* 31(6): 873–84.

Kawai, T. & Akira, S. (2009). The roles of tlrs, rlrs and nlrs in pathogen recognition, *Int Immunol* 21(4): 317–37.

Kawano, T., Cui, J., Koezuka, Y., Toura, I., Kaneko, Y., Motoki, K., Ueno, H., Nakagawa, R., Sato, H., Kondo, E., Koseki, H. & Taniguchi, M. (1997). Cd1d-restricted and tcr-mediated activation of valpha14 nkt cells by glycosylceramides, *Science* 278(5343): 1626–9.

Kinjo, Y., Tupin, E., Wu, D., Fujio, M., Garcia-Navarro, R., Benhnia, M. R., Zajonc, D. M., Ben-Menachem, G., Ainge, G. D., Painter, G. F., Khurana, A., Hoebe, K., Behar, S. M., Beutler, B., Wilson, I. A., Tsuji, M., Sellati, T. J., Wong, C. H. & Kronenberg, M. (2006). Natural killer t cells recognize diacylglycerol antigens from pathogenic bacteria, *Nat. Immunol.* 7(9): 978–86.

Klinman, D. M., Yi, A. K., Beaucage, S. L., Conover, J. & Krieg, A. M. (1996). Cpg motifs present in bacteria dna rapidly induce lymphocytes to secrete interleukin 6, interleukin 12, and interferon gamma, *Proc Natl Acad Sci U S A* 93(7): 2879–83.

Kumar, H., Belperron, A., Barthold, S. W. & Bockenstedt, L. K. (2000). Cutting edge: Cd1d deficiency impairs murine host defense against the spirochete, borrelia burgdorferi, *J. Immunol.* 165(9): 4797–801.

Kurimoto, T., Suzuki, M. & Watanabe, T. (1990). [chemical composition and biological activities of lipopolysaccharides extracted from treponema denticola and treponema vincentii], *Shigaku* 78(2): 208–32.

Leadbetter, E. A., Brigl, M., Illarionov, P., Cohen, N., Luteran, M. C., Pillai, S., Besra, G. S. & Brenner, M. B. (2008). Nk t cells provide lipid antigen-specific cognate help for b cells, *Proc Natl Acad Sci U S A* 105(24): 8339–44.

Lien, E., Sellati, T. J., Yoshimura, A., Flo, T. H., Rawadi, G., Finberg, R. W., Carroll, J. D., Espevik, T., Ingalls, R. R., Radolf, J. D. & Golenbock, D. T. (1999). Toll-like receptor 2 functions as a pattern recognition receptor for diverse bacterial products, *J. Biol. Chem.* 274(47): 33419–25.

Livermore, B. P., Bey, R. F. & Johnson, R. C. (1978). Lipid metabolism of borrelia hermsi, *Infect. Immun.* 20(1): 215–20.

Livermore, B. P. & Johnson, R. C. (1970). Isolation and characterization of a glycolipid from treponema pallidum, kazan 5, *Biochim. Biophys. Acta* 210(2): 315–8.

Livermore, B. P. & Johnson, R. C. (1975). The lipids of four unusual non-pathogenic host-associated spirochetes, *Can. J. Microbiol.* 21(11): 1877–80.

Madan Babu, M. & Sankaran, K. (2002). Dolop–database of bacterial lipoproteins, *Bioinformatics* 18(4): 641–3.

Medzhitov, R., Preston-Hurlburt, P. & Janeway, C. A., J. (1997). A human homologue of the drosophila toll protein signals activation of adaptive immunity, *Nature* 388(6640): 394–7.

Moore, M. W., Cruz, A. R., LaVake, C. J., Marzo, A. L., Eggers, C. H., Salazar, J. C. & Radolf, J. D. (2007). Phagocytosis of borrelia burgdorferi and treponema pallidum potentiates innate immune activation and induces gamma interferon production, *Infect Immun* 75(4): 2046–62.

Morr, M., Takeuchi, O., Akira, S., Simon, M. M. & Muhlradt, P. F. (2002). Differential recognition of structural details of bacterial lipopeptides by toll-like receptors, *Eur. J. Immunol.* 32(12): 3337–47.

Norgard, M. V., Arndt, L. L., Akins, D. R., Curetty, L. L., Harrich, D. A. & Radolf, J. D. (1996). Activation of human monocytic cells by treponema pallidum and borrelia burgdorferi lipoproteins and synthetic lipopeptides proceeds via a pathway distinct from that of lipopolysaccharide but involves the transcriptional activator nf-kappa b, *Infect. Immun.* 64(9): 3845–52.

Norgard, M. V., Riley, B. S., Richardson, J. A. & Radolf, J. D. (1995). Dermal inflammation elicited by synthetic analogs of treponema pallidum and borrelia burgdorferi lipoproteins, *Infect Immun* 63(4): 1507–15.

Norris, S. J., Paster, B. J., Moter, A. & GA¶bel, U. B. (2006). The Genus Treponema, *in* M. Dworkin & S. Falkow (eds), *The Prokaryotes*, Vol. 7, Springer, New York, pp. 211–234.

Oosting, M., Berende, A., Sturm, P., Ter Hofstede, H. J., de Jong, D. J., Kanneganti, T. D., van der Meer, J. W., Kullberg, B. J., Netea, M. G. & Joosten, L. A. (2010). Recognition of borrelia burgdorferi by nod2 is central for the induction of an inflammatory reaction, *J Infect Dis* 201(12): 1849–58.

Opitz, B., SchrA¶der, N. W., Spreitzer, I., Michelsen, K. S., Kirschning, C. J., Hallatschek, W., Zähringer, U., Hartung, T., GA¶bel, U. B. & Schumann, R. R. (2001). Toll-like receptor-2 mediates treponema glycolipid and lipoteichoic acid-induced nf-kappab translocation, *J Biol Chem* 276(25): 22041–7.

Paster, B. J., Dewhirst, F. E., Weisburg, W. G., Tordoff, L. A., Fraser, G. J., Hespell, R. B., Stanton, T. B., Zablen, L., Mandelco, L. & Woese, C. R. (1991). Phylogenetic analysis of the spirochetes, *J. Bacteriol.* 173(19): 6101–9.

Penn, C. W., Cockayne, A. & Bailey, M. J. (1985). The outer membrane of treponema pallidum: biological significance and biochemical properties, *J Gen Microbiol* 131(9): 2349–57.

Petzke, M. M., Brooks, A., Krupna, M. A., Mordue, D. & Schwartz, I. (2009). Recognition of borrelia burgdorferi, the lyme disease spirochete, by tlr7 and tlr9 induces a type i ifn response by human immune cells, *J Immunol* 183(8): 5279–92.

Poltorak, A., He, X., Smirnova, I., Liu, M. Y., Van Huffel, C., Du, X., Birdwell, D., Alejos, E., Silva, M., Galanos, C., Freudenberg, M., Ricciardi-Castagnoli, P., Layton, B. & Beutler,

B. (1998). Defective lps signaling in c3h/hej and c57bl/10sccr mice: mutations in tlr4 gene, *Science* 282(5396): 2085–8.

Que-Gewirth, N. L., Ribeiro, A. A., Kalb, S. R., Cotter, R. J., Bulach, D. M., Adler, B., Girons, I. S., Werts, C. & Raetz, C. R. (2004). A methylated phosphate group and four amide-linked acyl chains in leptospira interrogans lipid a. the membrane anchor of an unusual lipopolysaccharide that activates tlr2, *J. Biol. Chem.* 279(24): 25420–9.

Qureshi, S. T., Lariviere, L., Leveque, G., Clermont, S., Moore, K. J., Gros, P. & Malo, D. (1999). Endotoxin-tolerant mice have mutations in toll-like receptor 4 (tlr4), *J Exp Med* 189(4): 615–25.

Radolf, J. D., Arndt, L. L., Akins, D. R., Curetty, L. L., Levi, M. E., Shen, Y., Davis, L. S. & Norgard, M. V. (1995). Treponema pallidum and borrelia burgdorferi lipoproteins and synthetic lipopeptides activate monocytes/macrophages, *J. Immunol.* 154(6): 2866–77.

Radolf, J. D., Chamberlain, N. R., Clausell, A. & Norgard, M. V. (1988). Identification and localization of integral membrane proteins of virulent treponema pallidum subsp. pallidum by phase partitioning with the nonionic detergent triton x-114, *Infect. Immun.* 56(2): 490–8.

Radolf, J. D. & Norgard, M. V. (1988). Pathogen specificity of treponema pallidum subsp. pallidum integral membrane proteins identified by phase partitioning with triton x-114, *Infect Immun* 56(7): 1825–8.

Radolf, J. D., Norgard, M. V., Brandt, M. E., Isaacs, R. D., Thompson, P. A. & Beutler, B. (1991). Lipoproteins of borrelia burgdorferi and treponema pallidum activate cachectin/tumor necrosis factor synthesis. analysis using a cat reporter construct, *J. Immunol.* 147(6): 1968–74.

Radolf, J. D., Norgard, M. V. & Schulz, W. W. (1989). Outer membrane ultrastructure explains the limited antigenicity of virulent treponema pallidum, *Proc Natl Acad Sci U S A* 86(6): 2051–5.

Radolf, J. D., Robinson, E. J., Bourell, K. W., Akins, D. R., Porcella, S. F., Weigel, L. M., Jones, J. D. & Norgard, M. V. (1995). Characterization of outer membranes isolated from treponema pallidum, the syphilis spirochete, *Infect. Immun.* 63(11): 4244–52.

Rosen, G., Sela, M. N., Naor, R., Halabi, A., Barak, V. & Shapira, L. (1999). Activation of murine macrophages by lipoprotein and lipooligosaccharide of treponema denticola, *Infect Immun* 67(3): 1180–6.

Ruby, J., Rehani, K. & Martin, M. (2007). Treponema denticola activates mitogen-activated protein kinase signal pathways through toll-like receptor 2, *Infect Immun* 75(12): 5763–8.

Schaudinn, F. R. & Hoffmann, E. (1905). Vorläufiger Bericht über das Vorkommen von Spirochaeten in syphilitischen Krankheitsprodukten und bei Papillomen, *Arbeiten aus dem Kaiserlichen Gesundheitsamte*, Vol. 22, Springer, Berlin, pp. 527–534.

Schröder, N. W., Heine, H., Alexander, C., Manukyan, M., Eckert, J., Hamann, L., Göbel, U. B. & Schumann, R. R. (2004). Lipopolysaccharide binding protein binds to triacylated and diacylated lipopeptides and mediates innate immune responses, *J. Immunol.* 173(4): 2683–91.

Schröder, N. W., Opitz, B., Lamping, N., Michelsen, K. S., Zähringer, U., Göbel, U. B. & Schumann, R. R. (2000). Involvement of lipopolysaccharide binding protein, cd14, and toll-like receptors in the initiation of innate immune responses by treponema glycolipids, *J. Immunol.* 165(5): 2683–93.

Schultz, C. P., Wolf, V., Lange, R., Mertens, E., Wecke, J., Naumann, D. & Zähringer, U. (1998). Evidence for a new type of outer membrane lipid in oral spirochete treponema denticola. functioning permeation barrier without lipopolysaccharides, *J. Biol. Chem.* 273(25): 15661–6.

Schumann, R. R., Leong, S. R., Flaggs, G. W., Gray, P. W., Wright, S. D., Mathison, J. C., Tobias, P. S. & Ulevitch, R. J. (1990). Structure and function of lipopolysaccharide binding protein, *Science* 249(4975): 1429–31.

Sellati, T. J., Bouis, D. A., Kitchens, R. L., Darveau, R. P., Pugin, J., Ulevitch, R. J., Gangloff, S. C., Goyert, S. M., Norgard, M. V. & Radolf, J. D. (1998). Treponema pallidum and borrelia burgdorferi lipoproteins and synthetic lipopeptides activate monocytic cells via a cd14-dependent pathway distinct from that used by lipopolysaccharide, *J. Immunol.* 160(11): 5455–64.

Seshadri, R., Myers, G. S., Tettelin, H., Eisen, J. A., Heidelberg, J. F., Dodson, R. J., Davidsen, T. M., DeBoy, R. T., Fouts, D. E., Haft, D. H., Selengut, J., Ren, Q., Brinkac, L. M., Madupu, R., Kolonay, J., Durkin, S. A., Daugherty, S. C., Shetty, J., Shvartsbeyn, A., Gebregeorgis, E., Geer, K., Tsegaye, G., Malek, J., Ayodeji, B., Shatsman, S., McLeod, M. P., Smajs, D., Howell, J. K., Pal, S., Amin, A., Vashisth, P., McNeill, T. Z., Xiang, Q., Sodergren, E., Baca, E., Weinstock, G. M., Norris, S. J., Fraser, C. M. & Paulsen, I. T. (2004). Comparison of the genome of the oral pathogen treponema denticola with other spirochete genomes, *Proc. Natl. Acad. Sci. USA* 101(15): 5646–51.

Setubal, J. C., Reis, M., Matsunaga, J. & Haake, D. A. (2006). Lipoprotein computational prediction in spirochaetal genomes, *Microbiology* 152(Pt 1): 113–21.

Shimazu, R., Akashi, S., Ogata, H., Nagai, Y., Fukudome, K., Miyake, K. & Kimoto, M. (1999). Md-2, a molecule that confers lipopolysaccharide responsiveness on toll-like receptor 4, *J Exp Med* 189(11): 1777–82.

Shin, O. S., Isberg, R. R., Akira, S., Uematsu, S., Behera, A. K. & Hu, L. T. (2008). Distinct roles for myd88 and toll-like receptors 2, 5, and 9 in phagocytosis of borrelia burgdorferi and cytokine induction, *Infect Immun* 76(6): 2341–51.

Smith, K. D., Andersen-Nissen, E., Hayashi, F., Strobe, K., Bergman, M. A., Barrett, S. L., Cookson, B. T. & Aderem, A. (2003). Toll-like receptor 5 recognizes a conserved site on flagellin required for protofilament formation and bacterial motility, *Nat Immunol* 4(12): 1247–53.

Stübs, G., Fingerle, V., Wilske, B., Göbel, U. B., Zähringer, U., Schumann, R. R. & Schröder, N. W. (2009). Acylated cholesteryl galactosides are specific antigens of borrelia causing lyme disease and frequently induce antibodies in late stages of disease, *J. Biol. Chem.* 284(20): 13326–34.

Subramanian, G., Koonin, E. V. & Aravind, L. (2000). Comparative genome analysis of the pathogenic spirochetes borrelia burgdorferi and treponema pallidum, *Infect. Immun.* 68(3): 1633–48.

Takada, H., Yokoyama, S. & Yang, S. (2002). Enhancement of endotoxin activity by muramyldipeptide, *J Endotoxin Res* 8(5): 337–42.

Takayama, K., Rothenberg, R. J. & Barbour, A. G. (1987). Absence of lipopolysaccharide in the lyme disease spirochete, borrelia burgdorferi, *Infect. Immun.* 55(9): 2311–3.

Takeuchi, O., Kawai, T., Muhlradt, P. F., Morr, M., Radolf, J. D., Zychlinsky, A., Takeda, K. & Akira, S. (2001). Discrimination of bacterial lipoproteins by toll-like receptor 6, *Int. Immunol.* 13(7): 933–40.

Takeuchi, O., Sato, S., Horiuchi, T., Hoshino, K., Takeda, K., Dong, Z., Modlin, R. L. & Akira, S. (2002). Cutting edge: role of toll-like receptor 1 in mediating immune response to microbial lipoproteins, *J. Immunol.* 169(1): 10–4.

Ting, J. P., Lovering, R. C., Alnemri, E. S., Bertin, J., Boss, J. M., Davis, B. K., Flavell, R. A., Girardin, S. E., Godzik, A., Harton, J. A., Hoffman, H. M., Hugot, J. P., Inohara, N., Mackenzie, A., Maltais, L. J., Nunez, G., Ogura, Y., Otten, L. A., Philpott, D., Reed, J. C., Reith, W., Schreiber, S., Steimle, V. & Ward, P. A. (2008). The nlr gene family: a standard nomenclature, *Immunity* 28(3): 285–7.

Tupin, E., Benhnia, M. R., Kinjo, Y., Patsey, R., Lena, C. J., Haller, M. C., Caimano, M. J., Imamura, M., Wong, C. H., Crotty, S., Radolf, J. D., Sellati, T. J. & Kronenberg, M. (2008). Nkt cells prevent chronic joint inflammation after infection with borrelia burgdorferi, *Proc. Natl. Acad. Sci. USA* 105(50): 19863–8.

Uematsu, S., Jang, M. H., Chevrier, N., Guo, Z., Kumagai, Y., Yamamoto, M., Kato, H., Sougawa, N., Matsui, H., Kuwata, H., Hemmi, H., Coban, C., Kawai, T., Ishii, K. J., Takeuchi, O., Miyasaka, M., Takeda, K. & Akira, S. (2006). Detection of pathogenic intestinal bacteria by toll-like receptor 5 on intestinal cd11c+ lamina propria cells, *Nat Immunol* 7(8): 868–74.

Umemoto, T., Ota, T., Sagawa, H., Kato, K., Takada, H., Tsujimoto, M., Kawasaki, A., Ogawa, T., Harada, K. & Kotani, S. (1981). Chemical and biological properties of a peptidoglycan isolated from treponema pallidum kazan, *Infect. Immun.* 31(2): 767–74.

Vinh, T., Adler, B. & Faine, S. (1986). Ultrastructure and chemical composition of lipopolysaccharide extracted from leptospira interrogans serovar copenhageni, *J. Gen. Microbiol.* 132(1): 103–9.

Viriyakosol, S., Kirkland, T., Soldau, K. & Tobias, P. (2000). Md-2 binds to bacterial lipopolysaccharide, *J Endotoxin Res* 6(6): 489–91.

Walker, E. M., Zampighi, G. A., Blanco, D. R., Miller, J. N. & Lovett, M. A. (1989). Demonstration of rare protein in the outer membrane of treponema pallidum subsp. pallidum by freeze-fracture analysis, *J Bacteriol* 171(9): 5005–11.

Walker, S. G., Xu, X., Altman, E., Davis, K. J., Ebersole, J. L. & Holt, S. C. (1999). Isolation and chemical analysis of a lipopolysaccharide from the outer membrane of the oral anaerobic spirochete treponema pectinovorum, *Oral Microbiol Immunol* 14(5): 304–8.

Wang, J. E., Jorgensen, P. F., Ellingsen, E. A., Almiof, M., Thiemermann, C., Foster, S. J., Aasen, A. O. & Solberg, R. (2001). Peptidoglycan primes for lps-induced release of proinflammatory cytokines in whole human blood, *Shock* 16(3): 178–82.

Werts, C., Tapping, R. I., Mathison, J. C., Chuang, T. H., Kravchenko, V., Saint Girons, I., Haake, D. A., Godowski, P. J., Hayashi, F., Ozinsky, A., Underhill, D. M., Kirschning, C. J., Wagner, H., Aderem, A., Tobias, P. S. & Ulevitch, R. J. (2001). Leptospiral lipopolysaccharide activates cells through a tlr2-dependent mechanism, *Nat. Immunol.* 2(4): 346–52.

Wright, S. D., Ramos, R. A., Tobias, P. S., Ulevitch, R. J. & Mathison, J. C. (1990). Cd14, a receptor for complexes of lipopolysaccharide (lps) and lps binding protein, *Science* 249(4975): 1431–3.

Yanagihara, Y., Kamisango, K., Yasuda, S., Kobayashi, S., Mifuchi, I., Azuma, I., Yamamura, Y. & Johnson, R. C. (1984). Chemical compositions of cell walls and polysaccharide fractions of spirochetes, *Microbiol. Immunol.* 28(5): 535–44.

2

Whole Genome Analyses of Treponemes: New Targets for Strain- and Subspecies-Specific Molecular Diagnostics

David Šmajs[1], Lenka Mikalová[1], Darina Čejková[1], Michal Strouhal[1], Marie Zobaníková[1], Petra Pospíšilová[1], Steven J. Norris[2] and George M. Weinstock[3]

[1]Masaryk University Czech Republic
[2]University of Texas-Houston Medical School
[3]Washington University School of Medicine
USA

1. Introduction

The genus *Treponema* comprises several human uncultivable pathogens including *Treponema pallidum* subspecies *pallidum* (TPA, the causative agent of the sexually transmitted syphilis), *Treponema pallidum* subspecies *pertenue* (TPE, causative agent of yaws), *Treponema pallidum* subspecies *endemicum* (TEN, causing endemic syphilis), and *Treponema carateum* causing pinta. Additionally, the rabbit pathogen *Treponema paraluiscuniculi* (TPC) is very similar to syphilis treponeme but is not pathogenic to humans. Other pathogenic treponemes (e.g. *Treponema denticola* and *T. vincentii*) differ from the others by having considerably larger genomes (MacDougall & Girons, 1995; Seshadri *et al.*, 2004). Moreover, these treponemes can be cultivated under *in vitro* conditions. The infections caused by human uncultivable pathogenic treponemes can be classified according to their invasivity, from the most invasive bacterium causing venereal syphilis to *Treponema carateum* (pinta), which is a non-invasive spirochete causing local dermal lesions (Antal *et al.*, 2002). Strains of non-venereal treponemes including *Treponema pallidum* subspecies *pertenue* and *endemicum* are considered moderately invasive.

The whole genome analyses of treponemes started with the completion of the whole genome sequence of *T. pallidum*, by Nichols strain in 1998 (Fraser *et al.*, 1998). Since then, a number of genome studies have been performed (e.g. Brinkmann *et al.*, 2006; Giacani *et al.*, 2010; Harper *et al.*, 2008a; Matějková *et al.*, 2008; McKevitt *et al.*, 2003; McKevitt *et al.*, 2005; Mikalová *et al.*, 2010; Šmajs *et al.*, 2005; Strouhal *et al.*, 2007; Titz *et al.*, 2008). The genomic data has provided new opportunities to study pathogenic treponemes and increase our understanding of these unique pathogens.

Serological tests are considered standard laboratory methods for the diagnosis of syphilis since direct diagnostic methods are limited by the fact that the *T. pallidum* treponemes cannot be cultured continuously under *in vitro* conditions. The rabbit infectivity test (RIT) is the gold standard for demonstrating *T. pallidum* infection, but is impractical for clinical use because of high costs and delayed test results. Microscopic identification of treponemes in clinical samples, particularly in combination with direct fluorescent antibody tests using anti-*T. pallidum* antibodies, is highly specific for treponemal infections; however, it does not distinguish between pathogenic treponemal species and requires technical expertise that is not commonly available in a clinical setting. Observed clinical manifestations, history, and serology have thus been the standard procedure for diagnosis of treponemal infections for the past century. However, the available serologic tests have several important limitations: i) the antibody response to treponemal infections is often not detectable during the first 1-3 weeks of infection, ii) routine treponemal tests for syphilis, which detect IgG antibodies, will be positive if the patient has a previous history of syphilitic infections, iii) diagnosis of congenital syphilis can be confused by transferred antibodies from the mother, and iv) serological tests in patients with a risk of endemic treponematoses cannot distinguish between these infections and syphilis.

In the last years, there has been an increasing effort to apply PCR techniques for direct diagnosis of syphilis (for review see Šmajs *et al.*, 2006). PCR detection of treponemal DNA is a direct method with sensitivity as low as a few copies of the treponemal chromosome per PCR reaction. Moreover, PCR detection of treponemal 16S rRNA, present in many copies per single treponemal genome increases the sensitivity to 10^{-2} - 10^{-3} genome equivalents (Centurion-Lara *et al.*, 1997). However, the relatively low numbers of treponemes in whole blood put limitations on PCR diagnosis of syphilis from blood samples.

2. Whole genome analyses of uncultivable treponemes

2.1 Whole genome fingerprinting

The genomes of nine uncultivable treponemes including *T. p. pallidum* strains (Nichols, SS14, DAL-1 and Mexico A), *T. p. pertenue* strains (Samoa D, CDC-2 and Gauthier), *Treponema paraluiscuniculi* Cuniculi A strain, and the Fribourg-Blanc simian isolate, were studied using the whole genome fingerprinting technique (WGF, Mikalová *et al.*, 2010; Strouhal *et al.*, 2007; Weinstock *et al.*, 2000). More than 130 individual amplicons covering the entire genome were digested with a set of several restriction endonucleases and the resulting restriction fragments were visualized using gel electrophoresis. WGF was used to estimate the genome size, genome structure and the sequentially diverse chromosomal regions (Table 1).

The observed differences, in the presence of restriction target sites, grouped *T. p. pallidum* strains into a separate cluster compared to *T. p. pertenue* strains. The Fribourg-Blanc isolate, although more distantly separated, was clustered with TPE strains (Fig. 1). Analysis of the *tpr*C and *tpr*I gene phylogeny (Gray *et al.*, 2006) revealed similar close relationships between the Fribourg-Blanc treponemes and *T. p. pertenue* strains. The Fribourg-Blanc isolate is infectious to humans and is able to cause symptoms of yaws (Smith, 1971; Smith *et al.*, 1971). Although the genome analysis of *T. pallidum* ssp. *endemicum* strain Bosnia A (Grin, 1952) has not yet been completed, the preliminary analysis of more than a quarter of the genome (25.6%) has revealed a relatedness among the TEN Bosnia A strain, TPE strains, and the Fribourg-Blanc treponeme (Fig. 1, panel B). The observed relatedness between the TPE and the Fribourg-Blanc strains suggests a possible common origin of these strains and potentially indicates treponemal strain transmission between humans and African primates. Since yaws and simian treponemal infections occur in overlapping geographic territories, human treponemal pathogens may have originated in Africa (Livingstone, 1991). The observed restriction target site diversity among TPA strains indicates the presence of two separated groups (the Nichols group and the SS14 group) of TPA strains that coexist in the human population.

Strain name	Species/ Subspecies*	Place and year of isolation	Revealed genome size (kb)	Revealed genome sequence identity with Nichols (%)	Reference
Nichols	TPA	Washington, DC; 1912	1139.6†	100	Mikalová *et al.*, 2010; Nichols & Hough, 1913
DAL-1	TPA	Dallas; 1991	1139.9	99.98	Mikalová *et al.*, 2010; Wendel *et al.*, 1991
SS14	TPA	Atlanta; 1977	1139.5	99.92	Mikalová *et al.*, 2010; Stamm *et al.*, 1983
Mexico A	TPA	Mexico; 1953	1140.0	99.93	Turner & Hollander, 1957; Mikalová *et al.*, 2010
Samoa D	TPE	Western Samoa; 1953	1139.3	99.64	Turner & Hollander, 1957; Mikalová *et al.*, 2010
CDC-2	TPE	Akorabo, Ghana; 1980	1139.7	99.63	Liska *et al.*, 1982; Mikalová *et al.*, 2010
Gauthier	TPE	Congo; 1960	1139.4	99.64	Gastinel *et al.*, 1963; Mikalová *et al.*, 2010
Fribourg-Blanc	?	Guinea; 1966	1140.4	99.57	Fribourg-Blanc & Mollaret, 1969; Mikalová *et al.*, 2010
Cuniculi A	TPC	?	1133.4	98.21	Strouhal *et al.*, 2007

* TPA = T. pallidum subsp. pallidum; TPE = T. pallidum subsp. pertenue; TPC = T. paraluiscuniculi.
†The 1.2 kb tprK-like insertion in part of Nichols population (Šmajs et al., 2002) was added to the previously published genome sequence (Fraser et al., 1998).

Table 1. Genome size and revealed genome sequence identity with the Nichols genome of *T. p. pallidum*, *T. p. pertenue*, *T. paraluiscuniculi* and the Fribourg-Blanc strains.

The WGF technique also identified genomic regions showing variability in most investigated strains including the intergenic region between genes TP0126 and TP0127, and in the *arp*, TP0470, and TP0967 genes. Among the investigated TPA and TPE genomes, the *tpr*K-like sequence inserted between the TP0126 and TP0127 genes was found in three different versions (Mikalová *et al.*, 2010). In the Nichols genome, this insertion was found only in part of the treponemal population (Šmajs *et al.*, 2002). With regard to the *arp* gene

(Pillay *et al.*, 1998), a variable number of tandem repetitions were found in the tested genomes. Based on amino acid variations, previously published papers (Harper *et al.*, 2008b; Liu *et al.*, 2007) classified the TPA and TPE Arp repeat motifs into 4 types (I, II, III, II/III), and the variability in repeat sequence types correlated with the sexual transmission strategy (Harper *et al.*, 2008b). The differences among tested strains were also found in a number of 24 bp tandem repeats of TP0470, a gene encoding a hypothetical protein, and in indels present in the hypothetical TP0967 gene (Mikalová *et al.*, 2010). As with the *tpr*K-like insertion between the TP0126 and TP0127 genes, the number of 24 bp repetitions in TP0470 was reported to vary within individual bacterial isolates (Marra *et al.*, 2010).

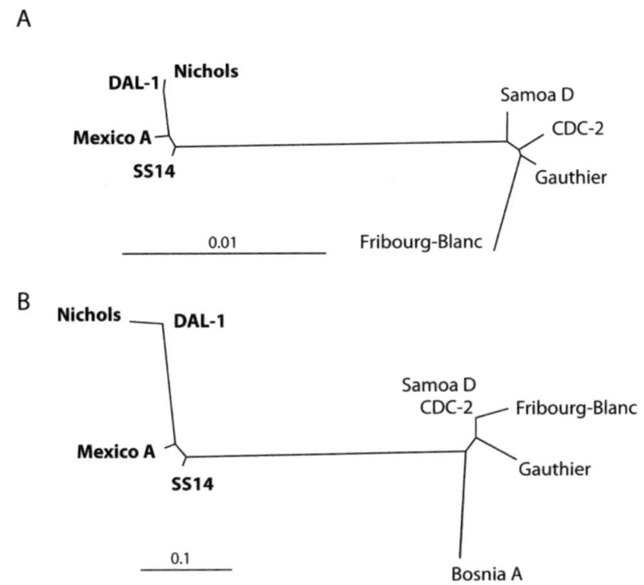

Fig. 1. Unrooted trees constructed from restriction target site data of the analyzed TPA and TPE genomes. Panel A: unrooted tree constructed from whole genome analyses. The Fribourg-Blanc isolate clusters with TPE strains. Panel B: unrooted tree constructed from 25.6% of the tested genomes. The Bosnia A strain clusters with TPE genomes, indicating a close relationship between this T. pallidum ssp. endemicum strain and TPE strains. The bar scale corresponds to 0.01 and 0.1 restriction target site (RTS) changes per RTS, respectively. TPA strains are shown in bold.

2.2 Whole genome sequencing

Historically, syphilis and yaws treponemes were considered to be separate species (based on differences in clinical manifestations of the corresponding diseases), but since 1984 they have been classified as subspecies (Smibert, 1984) based on DNA hybridization experiments (Miao and Fieldsteel, 1980).

The WGF technique revealed high sequence relatedness among all investigated genomes, with the most divergent, *T. paraluiscuniculi*, genome differing in less than 2% of the genome sequence (Strouhal *et al.*, 2007). These data indicated that complete, high-quality sequences were required for treponeme genome comparisons. The list of sequenced treponemal genomes and the status of sequencing is shown in Table 2.

With the exception of the Nichols and Chicago genomes, whole genome DNA sequencing has been performed using a combination of several approaches including comparative genome sequencing (CGS, Matějková *et al.*, 2008), 454 pyrosequencing (Margulies *et al.*, 2005) and the Solexa/Illumina method (Bennett, 2004). Isolated genomic DNA of most of the sequenced strains was amplified before genomic DNA sequencing. All discrepancies in CGS, 454 and Solexa/Illumina sequences were resequenced, using the dideoxyterminator sequencing method, until a final consensus sequence was obtained.

Treponemal strain	Treponeme	Sequencing method	Reference/GenBank accession number
Nichols	TPA	DDT	Fraser *et al.*, 1998
SS14	TPA	CGS	Matějková *et al.*, 2008
Chicago	TPA	Illumina	Giacani *et al.*, 2010
DAL-1	TPA	454, Illumina	unpublished
Mexico A	TPA	Illumina	unpublished
Samoa D	TPE	CGS, 454, Illumina	CP002374
CDC-2	TPE	454, Illumina	CP002375
Gauthier	TPE	454, Illumina	CP002376
Fribourg-Blanc	?	454, Illumina	unpublished
Cuniculi A	TPC	CGS, 454, Illumina	CP002103
Bosnia A	TEN	454, Illumina	unpublished

Table 2. Whole genome sequencing of uncultivable treponemal strains

Sequencing of the *T. paraluiscuniculi* genome revealed 99.16% sequence identity (Šmajs *et al.*, 2011) of the conserved regions of the Nichols and Cuniculi A genomes. The identity between TPA and TPE genomes, greater than 99.8%, was found during sequencing of three TPE genomes (Čejková *et al.*, unpublished data). In all sequenced genomes, no major genome rearrangements were found. Despite the different clinical manifestations and host specificities, a nearly identical gene order was found in TPA, TPE, and *T. paraluiscuniculi* strains, further establishing the close genetic relationship between these treponemal pathogens. The accuracy of genome assemblies and the sequencing error rate were estimated using the WGF approach and revealed high quality genome sequences with an error rate less than 10^{-4}. All investigated TPE strains were very similar in genome size with only 414 bp difference between the largest, CDC-2, and the smallest, Samoa D, genome. Nucleotide diversity (π) among sequenced TPE genomes was quite low (0.00032). In contrast, the nucleotide divergence (d_A) between TPA and TPE genomes was 3.6 - 4.6 times higher than the observed nucleotide diversity among each subspecies. These data indicate a significant evolutionary relationship between yaws and syphilis strains. Sequencing of additional TPA and TPE strains in the future will result in decreased numbers of genetic differences relevant to clinical manifestations of yaws and syphilis treponemes.

Altogether, 13 pseudogenes were found in the TPE genomes. In addition to pseudogenes, the genetic changes were analyzed in 970 similarly annotated protein-coding genes in both TPE and TPA strains. Compared to TPA strains, 70.4% of TPE genes encoded either identical proteins or identical proteins with strain specific differences; 194 (19.7%) genes encoded proteins with 1 amino acid substitution found in all tested TPE strains, 63 (6.4%) genes encoded proteins with 2 to 5 amino acid changes, and only 34 (3.5%) genes encoded proteins with 6 or more amino acid replacements or other major protein changes.

Major sequence changes between TPA and TPE treponemes were found in the sequence for ethanolaminephosphotransferase, which is a pseudogene in TPE strains (TPE_0671), and in additional 12 genes with predicted functions including 8 *tpr* genes. The Tpr proteins are heterogenous proteins considered as potential virulence factors involved in pathogenesis and/or immune evasion (Giacani *et al.*, 2004; Gray *et al.*, 2006), and in inducing an antibody response during treponemal infection (Centurion-Lara *et al.*, 1999, 2000a, 2000b). Other differences between TPA and TPE involved a Mcp (methyl-accepting chemotaxis protein, TPE_0488), three treponemal antigens (TPE_0136; (Brinkman *et al.*, 2008), the Tp92 - outer membrane protein (TPE_0326; Cameron *et al.*, 2000), the Arp protein (TPE_0433, Pillay *et al.*, 1998)) and an elongated RecQ protein (TPE_0103) (Čejková *et al.*, unpublished results).

3. Targets for TPA strain-specific molecular diagnostics

3.1 Multilocus analyses of treponemal strains

The whole genome analyses of treponemal genomes revealed chromosomal regions with accumulated genetic diversity between TPA and TPE strains (Fig. 2).

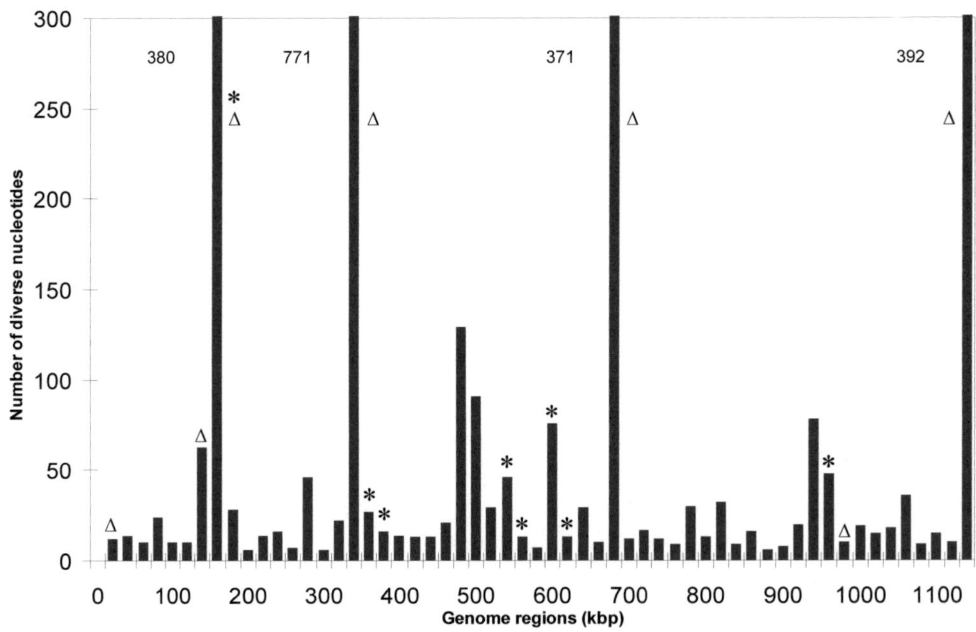

Fig. 2. Plot of numbers of nucleotide changes in 20 kb intervals between TPA and TPE strains along the treponemal chromosome. The exact number of nucleotide changes in the four most diverse regions is shown next to each column. Positions of selected chromosomal loci (see Table 3 and 4) are shown by asterisks. Positions of *tpr* genes in the treponemal genomes are shown with triangles (Δ).

In these regions, we determined the most genetically diverse genes and analyzed them in a set of TPA strains. In addition to four TPA strains (Nichols, SS14, DAL-1 and Mexico A),

TPA strains Grady (Atlanta, 1980), MN-3 (Minnesota, unknown), Philadelphia-1 (Philadelphia, 1988), Philadelphia-2 (Philadelphia, unknown), Bal-73-01 (Baltimore, 1973) were analyzed. All these strains were kindly provided by D. L. Cox, CDC, Atlanta, GA. The results of this analysis are summarized in the Tables 3 and 4. The greatest observed nucleotide difference was found in the TP0136 locus, followed by TP0548, TP0326 and TP0488. Interestingly, all investigated strains split into two subclusters containing either the Nichols or the SS14 strain (see Fig. 3).

	Differences in the nucleotide sequences, %, (difference in number of nt)			
Strain	TP0136	TP0326	TP0488	TP0548
Nichols	0	0	0	0
SS14	4.4	0.5	0.2	3.4
Mexico A	4.5	0.4	1.1	3.7
DAL-1	4.0	0 (0 nt)	0 (0 nt)	0 (0 nt)
Grady	4.4	0.5	0.1	3.4
MN-3	0.1	0 (1 nt)	0.1	0.8
Philadelphia 1	4.4	0.5	0.1	3.4
Philadelphia 2	0.1	0 (1 nt)	0.1	0.8
Bal-73-01	0 (0 nt)	0 (0 nt)	0 (1 nt)	0 (0 nt)

Table 3. Analysis of 4 chromosomal loci as potential targets for PCR detection and typing of clinical treponemal samples. The table shows the percentage of nucleotide differences compared to sequences present in the Nichols genome (Fraser *et al.*, 1998).

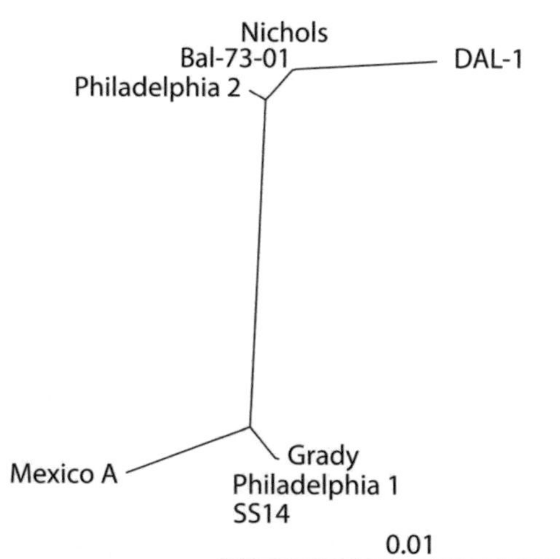

Fig. 3. The unrooted tree constructed from the nucleotide region resulting from concatenation of TP0136, TP0326, TP0488, and TP0548 loci sequenced in several TPA strains (of lengths ranging from 8342 to 8412 nucleotides). The bar scale corresponds to 0.01 nt changes per site. Please note that the TPA strains subcluster into two groups, one associated with the Nichols and the second associated with the SS14 strain.

In addition to TP0136, TP0548, TP0326 and TP0488 loci, we also tested other candidate chromosomal regions including TP0346, TP0515, TP0558, and TP0868 genes. The observed nucleotide diversity of these loci is shown in Table 4. The nucleotide diversity was considerably smaller among the latter group of genes (TP0346, TP0515, TP0558, and TP0868) indicating that their potential for testing of clinical TPA samples is lower than that of loci shown in Table 3. As in the previous case, Nichols-like strains were extremely similar to each other and distinct from SS14-like strains, reflecting different evolutionary relationships between these strains.

	Number of detected nucleotide changes			
Strain	TP0346	TP0515	TP0558	TP0868
Nichols	0	0	0	0
SS14	nd*	10	5	9
Mexico A	nd	nd	nd	2
DAL-1	0	0	0	0
Grady	2	nd	5	9
MN-3	0	nd	nd	0
Philadelphia 1	2	10	5	2
Philadelphia 2	nd	nd	nd	0
Bal-73-01	0	0	0	0

*nd, not determined

Table 4. Analysis of chromosomal loci as potential targets for PCR detection and typing of treponemes. The table shows the number of detected nucleotide changes compared to sequences present in the Nichols genome (Fraser *et al.*, 1998).

3.2 PCR analyses of clinical samples

Chromosomal genes including TP0136, TP0326, TP0488, TP0548, and TP0868, previously sequenced in TPA type strains, were used as DNA amplification targets from clinical samples containing treponemal DNA. The tested clinical samples were collected in the Czech Republic between years 2004 and 2010. The detected numbers of nucleotide changes were considerably lower than among the tested TPA type strains, indicating a genetic homogeneity of syphilis-causing strains in the Czech Republic. At locus TP0868, no diversity was observed among 5 tested clinical samples (see Table 5) and all TP0868 gene sequences were identical to the SS14 sequence. Interestingly, only strains identical or very similar to the SS14 strain were found among all investigated clinical strains (taken from 91 patients with sequenced treponemal DNA; unpublished results). Although not all gene sequences in the investigated strains were determined, the number of identified unique sequences (shown as unique a – d; Table 5) correlated with the number of nucleotide changes observed in Table 3, indicating that the most variable chromosomal regions identified during whole genome analyses were also the most variable among sequentially related clinical strains, i.e. causing syphilis, from particular geographic areas.

Clinical sample	TP0136	TP0548	TP0326	TP0488	TP0868	23S rDNA	No. of repetitions in the *arp* gene	*tpr*EGJ genes
D-151	unique a*	SS14-like	nd**	nd	SS14-like	sensitive***	8	d****
3Z	unique b	SS14-like	nd	nd	nd	sensitive	14	d
2K	SS14-like	unique a	nd	nd	nd	A2058G	14	d
G-269	SS14-like	unique b	nd	nd	SS14-like	sensitive	14	p
RL73	nd	unique c	nd	nd	nd	A2059G	nd	d
1Z	nd	unique d	nd	nd	nd	A2058G	14	d
50AZ	SS14-like	nd	unique a	unique a	SS14-like	A2059G	15	d
11379	SS14-like	nd	SS14-like	unique a	SS14-like	sensitive	11	d
24K	SS14-like	SS14-like	nd	nd	nd	sensitive	14	d
40K	SS14-like	SS14-like	nd	nd	nd	A2058G	14	d
8284	SS14-like	SS14-like	nd	nd	nd	A2059G	15	d
24AZ	SS14-like	SS14-like	nd	nd	nd	A2059G	12	d
37K	nd	nd	nd	nd	nd	A2058G	12	d
No. of different genotypes	3	5	2	1	1	3	5	2

*unique a, sequencing of this locus revealed a sequence different from the SS14 sequence. Different sequences at a particular locus are denoted with letters a-d.
**nd, not determined
***sensitive, unmutated 23S rRNA resulting in susceptibility of TPA strains to macrolide antibiotics; A2058G or A2059G mutations result in resistance to macrolides.
****d, restriction patterns according to Pillay et al., (1998)

Table 5. Analysis of chromosomal loci as potential targets for PCR detection and typing of treponemes. Data for 13 selected samples isolated between the 2004 and 2010 from patients in Czech Republic are shown.

The data shown in Table 5 indicate numbers of different genotypes identified by sequencing analysis of several treponemal chromosomal loci. The greatest numbers of genotypes were found for the locus TP0548 (5) and for genetic variants detected by amplification of the *arp* gene (5). The use of the TP0548 locus in molecular typing of syphilis was first described by Flasarová *et al.* (2006) and this locus was recently incorporated to the enhanced molecular typing system of *Treponema pallidum* (Marra *et al.*, 2010). Analysis of TP0136 revealed 3 genotypes. Although the loci TP0326, TP0488 and TP0868 were sequenced in only a few of the presented isolates, one to two different genotypes were identified. Moreover, the unique sequences for the investigated TP loci appear to vary independently with each other and also vary independently with the number of repetitions in the *arp* gene and restriction profile of *tpr*EGJ genes. This finding indicates the potential of using the above stated chromosomal loci in a detailed genetic identification of clinical samples. Although the typing of 23S rDNA locus revealed three genotypes, one encoding sensitivity to macrolide antibiotics and two coding for macrolide resistance (A2058G and A2059G mutations, respectively; Lukehart *et al.*, 2004; Matějková *et al.*, 2009; Stamm & Bergen, 2000), their use in molecular typing is probably limited by the fact that these mutations can be selected by use of macrolide antibiotics in a population. In the Czech Republic, more than 35% of clinical samples were found to contain a mutation encoding resistance to macrolide antibiotics (Flasarová *et al.*, unpublished results). In contrast, screening of 23S rDNA for A2058G in syphilitic samples taken from patients in Madagascar revealed no such mutation in 141 samples (Van Damme *et al.*, 2009). The recently improved CDC typing system (Marra *et al.*, 2010) relies on detection of the number of repetitions in the *arp* gene, on amplification and restriction digest analysis of *tpr*EGJ genes and on sequencing of a part of the TP0548 gene.

4. Chromosomal targets for detection of non-TPA strains

4.1 Chromosomal targets for detection of TPE strains

Endemic treponematoses (caused by *T. pallidum* subsp. *pertenue*, *T. pallidum* subsp. *endemicum* and *T. carateum*) are estimated to currently affect more than 2.5 million people worldwide (Antal *et al.*, 2002). In the previous century, the number of yaws cases decreased from 50 million to a few million. In recent years, yaws has re-emerged in several rural populations in Africa, Asia and South America and a new effort to eradicate this disease has recently been undertaken (Asiedu *et al.*, 2008). Since single-dose penicillin is both cheap and available and no other disease reservoirs (besides humans and primates) are known, the chances for yaws eradication are relatively good. Molecular diagnosis of yaws treponemes in this situation is of fundamental importance. In the last two decades, several subtle genetic differences between TPA and TPE strains were published (Walker *et al.*, 1995; Centurion-Lara *et al.*, 1998; Centurion-Lara *et al.*, 2006). The most prominent indels common for all investigated TPE strains are shown in Table 6.

The regions listed in Table 6 and several additional regions (Mikalová *et al.*, 2010) need to be tested for other TPE strains before selecting the most suitable target for a molecular diagnosis of the yaws causing strains. Interestingly, all these indels are also found in the Fribourg-Blanc genome. However, the Fribourg-Blanc isolate can be differentiated based on the presence of specific indels (Mikalová *et al.*, 2010) as well as other individual TPE strains (Mikalová *et al.*, 2010).

Intergenic region (IGR) or gene(s)	Detected indel (bp)	GenBank accession no.
TP0266 (278334-278366)*	deletion (33 bp)	HM165228 Samoa D HM165229 Gauthier HM165230 CDC-2 HM165231 Fribourg-Blanc
TP0316 (331265-331266)	insertion (635 bp)	HM585230 Samoa D HM585231 Gauthier HM585232 CDC-2 HM585233 Fribourg-Blanc
IGR TP0548-TP0549 (593023-593024)	insertion (52 bp)	HM245777 Samoa D HM243496 Gauthier HM243495 CDC-2 HM585227 Fribourg-Blanc
TP1030-TP1031 (1123987-1124363)	deletion (377 bp)	HM623430 Samoa D HM585235 Gauthier HM585236 CDC-2 HM585254 Fribourg-Blanc

*The coordinates refer to the published Nichols genome (Fraser et al., 1998)

Table 6. Most prominent indels identified in all investigated TPE strains (Samoa D, CDC-2, and Gauthier). All these changes were also found in the Fribourg-Blanc genome (Mikalová *et al.*, 2010).

4.2 Chromosomal targets for detection of TEN strains

The ongoing whole genome sequencing project of *T. p. endemicum* strain Bosnia A has already identified indels in at least 4 regions (ranging between 13 and ~60 bp), which can be used to differentiate the bejel treponeme from both the *T. p. pallidum* and *T. p. pertenue* strains (Table 7).

Intergenic region (IGR) or gene(s)	Detected indel (bp)	Coordinates in the Samoa D genome* (GenBank accession no. CP002374)
IGR TP0085-TP0086	deletion (13 bp)	94986-94998
TP0136	insertion (~0,06 kbp)	158205-158206
TP0326	insertion (15 bp)	348027-348028
TP0865	deletion (~25 bp)	945694-945718

*positions of detected indels in the TEN Bosnia A genome are shown as coordinates thereof in the Samoa D genome (GenBank accession no. CP002374)

Table 7. Indels identified in the TEN Bosnia A strain when compared to other investigated TPA and TPE strains.

5. Conclusions

The genomes of 9 pathogenic treponemes including *T. p. pallidum* strains (Nichols, SS14, DAL-1 and Mexico A), *T. p. pertenue* strains (Samoa D, CDC-2 and Gauthier), the Fribourg-Blanc isolate and *T. p. endemicum* (Bosnia A) were analyzed using several approaches including whole genome fingerprinting and whole genome sequencing. Genome analyses revealed several important chromosomal loci suitable for diagnostic purposes including: i) syphilis-causing treponemes and their molecular typing, ii) yaws treponemes, and iii) bejel treponemes.

A sequencing-based typing scheme using simultaneous analysis of 3 loci (TP0136, TP0548 and 23S rDNA genes) in the *T. p. pallidum* genome was also evaluated. In addition, amplification of 23S rDNA locus and its subsequent restriction target analysis was used to detect mutations leading to macrolide resistance. The unique sequences in the investigated TP loci appear to combine independently with each other and also combine independently with the number of repetitions in the *arp* gene and restriction profiles of *tpr*EGJ genes. Several genomic regions were found to differ between *T. p. pallidum* and *T. p. pertenue* strains and comprised indels ranging from 33 bp in the TP0266 gene to 635 bp in the *tpr*F gene (TP0316). In all cases, the Fribourg-Blanc simian isolate showed changes similar to *T. p. pertenue* strains suggesting a close relationship to the *pertenue* subspecies. A partial genome analysis of *T. p. endemicum* strain, Bosnia A, showed, that this strain clustered with TPE strains, though more distantly than that of the Fribourg-Blanc isolate. The Bosnia A genome contained indels in at least 4 regions (ranging between 13 and ~60 bp) that can be used to differentiate the bejel treponeme from both *T. p. pallidum* and *T. p. pertenue* strains.

6. Acknowledgements

The authors thank Dr. David Cox for providing several TPA and TPE type strains. The TEN Bosnia A strain was kindly provided by S. Bruisten. This work was supported by grants from the U.S. Public Health Service to G.M.W. (R01 DE12488 and R01 DE13759), and S.J.N. (R01 AI49252 and R03 AI69107) and by grants of the Grant Agency of the Czech Republic (310/07/0321), of the Ministry of Health of the Czech Republic (NT11159-5/2010), and the Ministry of Education of the Czech Republic (VZ MSM0021622415) to D.S.

7. References

Antal, G.M., Lukehart, S.A. & Meheus, A.Z. (2002). The endemic treponematoses. *Microbes and Infection*, Vol.4, No.1, (January 2002), pp. 83-94, ISSN 1286-4579

Asiedu, K., Amouzou, B. & Dhariwal, A. (2008). Yaws eradication: past efforts and future perspectives. *Bulletin of the World Health Organization*, Vol.86, No.7, (July 2008), pp. 499, ISSN 0042-9686

Bennett, S. (2004). Solexa Ltd. *Pharmacogenomics*, Vol.5, No.4, (June 2004), pp. 433–438, ISSN 1462-2416

Brinkman, M.B., McKevitt, M. & McLoughlin, M. (2006). Reactivity of antibodies from syphilis patients to a protein array representing the *Treponema pallidum* proteome. *Journal of Clinical Microbiology*, Vol.44, No.3, (March 2006), pp. 888-891, ISSN 0095-1137

Brinkman, M.B., McGill, M.A. & Pettersson, J.T. (2008). A novel *Treponema pallidum* antigen, TP0136, is an outer membrane protein that binds human fibronectin. *Infection and Immunity*, Vol.76, No.5, (May 2008), pp. 1848-1857, ISSN 0019-9567

Cameron, C.E., Lukehart, S.A. & Castro, C. (2000). Opsonic potential, protective capacity, and sequence conservation of the *Treponema pallidum* subspecies *pallidum* Tp92. *The*

Journal of Infectious Diseases, Vol.181, No.4, (April 2000), pp. 1401-1413, ISSN 0022-1899

Centurion-Lara, A., Castro, C. & Barrett, L. (1999). *Treponema pallidum* major sheath protein homologue TprK is a target of opsonic antibody and the protective immune response. *The Journal of Experimental Medicine,* Vol.189, No.4, (February 1999), pp.647-656, ISSN 0022-1007

Centurion-Lara, A., Castro, C. & Castillo, R. (1998). The flanking region sequences of the 15-kDa lipoprotein gene differentiate pathogenic treponemes. *The Journal of Infectious Diseases,* Vol.177, No.4, (April 1998), pp. 1036-1040, ISSN 0022-1899

Centurion-Lara, A., Castro, C. & Shaffer, J.M. (1997). Detection of *Treponema pallidum* by a sensitive reverse transcriptase PCR. *Journal of Clinical Microbiology,* Vol. 35, No. 6, (June 1997), pp. 1348-1352, ISSN 0095-1137

Centurion-Lara, A., Godornes, C. & Castro, C. (2000b). The *tpr*K gene is heterogeneous among *Treponema pallidum* strains and has multiple alleles. *Infection and Immunity,* Vol.68, No.2, (February 2000), pp. 824-831, ISSN 0019-9567

Centurion-Lara, A., Molini, B.J. & Godornes, C. (2006). Molecular differentiation of *Treponema pallidum* subspecies. *Journal of Clinical Microbiology* Vol.44, No.9, (September 2006), pp. 3377–3380, ISSN 0095-1137

Centurion-Lara, A., Sun, E.S. & Barrett, L.K. (2000a). Multiple alleles of *Treponema pallidum* repeat gene D in *Treponema pallidum* isolates. *Journal of Bacteriology,* Vol.182, No.8, (January 2000), pp. 2332-2335, ISSN 0021-9193

Flasarová, M., Šmajs, D. & Matějková, P. (2006). Molecular detection and subtyping of *Treponema pallidum* subsp. *pallidum* in clinical specimens. *Epidemiologie, mikrobiologie, imunologie,* Vol.55, No.3, (August 2006), pp. 105-111, ISSN 1210-7913

Fraser, C.M., Norris, S.J. & Weinstock, G.M. (1998). Complete genome sequence of *Treponema pallidum,* the syphilis spirochete. *Science,* Vol.281, No.5375, (July 1998), pp. 375-388, ISSN 0036-8075

Fribourg-Blanc, A., Mollaret, H.H. (1969). Natural treponematosis of the African primate. *Primates in medicine,* Vol.3, (n.d.), pp. 113-121

Gastinel, P., Vaisman, A. & Hamelin, A. (1963). Study of a recently isolated strain of *Treponema pertenue. La Prophylaxie sanitaire et morale.,* Vol.35, (July 1963), pp. 182-188

Giacani, L., Jeffrey, B.M. & Molini, B.J. (2010). Complete genome sequence and annotation of the *Treponema pallidum* subsp. *pallidum* Chicago strain. *Journal of Bacteriology,* Vol.192, No.10, (May 2010), pp. 2645-2646, ISSN 0021-9193

Giacani, L., Sun, E.S. & Hevner, K. (2004). Tpr homologs in *Treponema paraluiscuniculi* Cuniculi A strain. *Infection and Immunity,* Vol.72, No.11, (November 2004), pp. 6561-6576, ISSN 0019-9567

Gray, R.R., Mulligan, C.J. & Molini, B.J. (2006). Molecular evolution of the *tpr*C, D, I, K, G and J genes in the pathogenic genus *Treponema. Molecular Biology and Evolution,* Vol.23, No.11, (August 2006), pp. 2220-2233, ISSN 0737-4038

Grin, E.I. (1952). Endemic syphilis in Bosnia; clinical and epidemiological observations on a successful mass-treatment campaign. *Bulletin of the World Health Organization,* Vol.7, No.1, (n.d.), pp. 1-74, ISSN 0042-9686

Harper, K.N., Ocampo, P.S. & Steiner, B.M. (2008a). On the origin of the treponematoses: a phylogenetic approach. *PLoS Neglected Tropical Diseases,* Vol.2, No.1, (November 2007), pp. e148, ISSN 1935-2735

Harper, K.N., Liu, H. & Ocampo, P.S. (2008b). The sequence of the acidic repeat protein (*arp*) gene differentiates venereal from nonvenereal *Treponema pallidum* subspecies, and the gene has evolved under strong positive selection in the subspecies that causes syphilis. *FEMS Immunology and Medical Microbiology*, Vol.53, No.3, (August 2008), pp. 322-332, ISSN 1574-695X

Liska, S.L., Perine, P.L. & Hunter, E.F. (1982). Isolation and transportation of *Treponema pertenue* in golden hamsters. *Current Microbiology*, Vol.7, No.1, (n.d.), pp. 41-43, ISSN 0343-8651

Liu, H., Rodes, B. & George, R. (2007). Molecular characterization and analysis of a gene encoding the acidic repeat protein (Arp) of *Treponema pallidum*. *Journal of Medical Microbiology*, Vol.56, No.6, (June 2007), pp. 715-721, ISSN 0022-2615

Livingstone, F.B. (1991). On the origin of syphilis: an alternative hypothesis. *Current Anthropology*, Vol.32, No.5, (December 1991), pp. 587–590, ISSN 0011-3204

Lukehart, S.A., Godornes, C. & Molini, B.J. (2004). Macrolide resistance in *Treponema pallidum* in the United States and Ireland. *New England Journal of Medicine*, Vol.351, No.2, (July 2004), pp. 154–158, ISSN 0028-4793

MacDougall, J. & Saint Girons, I. (1995). Physical map of the *Treponema denticola* circular chromosome. *Journal of Bacteriology*, Vol.177, No.7, (April 1995), pp. 805-811, ISSN 0021-9193

Margulies, M., Egholm, M. & Altman, W.E. (2005). Genome sequencing in microfabricated high-density picolitre reactors. *Nature*, Vol.437, No.7057, (September 2005), pp. 376-380, ISSN 0028-0836.

Marra, Ch.M., Sahi, S.K. & Tantalo, L.C. (2010). Enhanced molecular typing of *Treponema pallidum*: geographical distribution of strain types and association with neurosyphilis. *Journal of Infectious Diseases*, Vol.202, No.9, (May 2010), pp. 1380-1388, ISSN 0022-1899

Matějková, P., Strouhal, M. & Šmajs, D. (2008). Complete genome sequence of *Treponema pallidum* ssp. *pallidum* strain SS14 determined with oligonucleotide arrays. *BMC Microbiology*, Vol.8, No.1, (n.d.), pp. 76, ISSN 1471-2180

Matějková, P., Flasarová, M. & Zákoucká, H. (2009). Macrolide treatment failure in a case of secondary syphilis: a novel A2059G mutation in the 23S rRNA gene of *Treponema pallidum* subsp. *pallidum*. *Journal of Medical Microbiology*, Vol.58, No.6, (June 2009), pp. 832-836, ISSN 0022-2615

McKevitt, M., Patel, K. & Šmajs, D. (2003). Systematic cloning of *Treponema pallidum* open reading frames for protein expression and antigen discovery. *Genome Research*, Vol.13, No.7, (July 2003); pp. 1665-1674, ISSN 1088-9051

McKevitt, M., Brinkman, M.B. & McLoughlin, M. (2005). Genome scale identification of *Treponema pallidum* antigens. *Infection and Immunity*, Vol.73, No.7, (July 2005), pp. 4445-4450, ISSN 0019-9567

Miao, R.M. & Fieldsteel, A.H. (1980). Genetic relationship between *Treponema pallidum* and *Treponema pertenue*, two noncultivable human pathogens. *Journal of Bacteriology*, Vol. 141, No. 1, (n.d.), pp. 427–429, ISSN 0021-9193

Mikalová, L., Strouhal, M. & Čejková, D. (2010). Genome analysis of *Treponema pallidum* subsp. *pallidum* and subsp. *pertenue* strains: Most of the genetic differences are localized in six regions. *PLoS One*, Vol.5, (December 2010), pp. e15713, ISSN 1932-6203

Nichols, H.J. & Hough, W.H. (1913). Demonstration of *Spirochaeta pallida* in the cerebrospinal fluid. *Journal of the American Medical Association*,Vol.60, No.2, (n.d.), pp. 108–110, ISSN 0002-9955

Pillay, A., Liu, H. & Chen, C.Y. (1998). Molecular subtyping of *Treponema pallidum* subspecies *pallidum*. *Sexually Transmitted Diseases*, Vol.25, No.8, (September 1998), pp. 408-414, ISSN 0148-5717

Seshadri, R., Myers, G.S.A. & Tettelin, H. (2004). Comparison of the genome of the oral pathogen *Treponema denticola* with other spirochete genomes. *PNAS*, Vol.101, No.15, (April 2004), pp. 5646–5651, ISSN 0027-8424

Šmajs, D., McKevitt, M. & Wang, L. (2002). BAC library of *T. pallidum* DNA in E. coli. *Genome Research*, Vol.12, No.3, (March 2002), pp. 515-522, ISSN 1088-9051

Šmajs, D., McKevitt, M. & Howell, J.K. (2005). Transcriptome of *Treponema pallidum*: gene expression profile during experimental rabbit infection. *Journal of Bacteriology*, Vol.187, No.5, (March 2005), pp. 1866-1874, ISSN 0021-9193

Šmajs, D., Matějková, P. & Woznicová, V. (2006). Diagnosis of syphilis by polymerase chain reaction and molecular typing of *Treponema pallidum*. *Reviews in Medical Microbiology*, Vol.17, No.4, (December 2006), pp. 93-100, ISSN 0954-139X

Šmajs, D., Zobaníková, M. & Strouhal, M. (2011). Complete genome sequence of *Treponema paraluiscuniculi*, strain Cuniculi A: the loss of infectivity to humans is associated with genome decay. *PLoS One*, Vol.6, No.5, (May 2011), pp. e20415, ISSN 1932-6203

Smibert, R.M. (1984). Genus III: *Treponema* Schaudinn 1905, 1728[AL], In: *Bergey's Manual of Systematic Bacteriology*, Krieg, N.R. & Holt, J.G., (Ed.), pp. 49-57, Williams&Wilkins, ISBN 0683041088, Baltimore, MD, USA

Smith, J.L. (1971). Neuro-ophthalmological study of late yaws. I. An introduction to yaws. *British Journal of Venereal Diseases and Genitourinary Medicine*, Vol.47, No.4, (January 1971), pp. 223–225

Smith, J.L., David, N.J. & Indgin, S. (1971). Neuro-ophthalmological study of late yaws and pinta. II. The Caracas project. *British Journal of Venereal Diseases and Genitourinary Medicine*, Vol.47, No.4, (January 1971), pp. 226–251

Stamm, L.V., Kerner, T.C. Jr & Bankaitis, V.A. (1983). Identification and preliminary characterization of *Treponema pallidum* protein antigens expressed in *Escherichia coli*. *Infection and Immunity*, Vol.41, No.2, (August 1983), pp. 709–721, ISSN 0019-9567

Stamm, L.V. & Bergen, H.L. (2000). A point mutation associated with bacterial macrolide resistance is present in both 23S rRNA genes of an erythromycin-resistant *Treponema pallidum* clinical isolate. *Antimicrobial Agents and Chemotherapy*, Vol.44, No.3, (Marz 2000), pp. 806–807, ISSN 0066-4804

Strouhal, M., Šmajs, D. & Matějková, P. (2007). Genome differences between *Treponema pallidum* subsp. *pallidum* strain Nichols and *T. paraluiscuniculi* strain Cuniculi A. *Infection and Immunity* , Vol.75, No.12, (December 2007), pp. 5859-5866, ISSN 0019-9567

Titz, B., Rajagopala, S.V. & Goll, J. (2008). The binary protein interactome of *Treponema pallidum*-the syphilis spirochete. *PLoS One*, Vol.3, No.5, (May 2008), pp. e2292, ISSN 1932-6203

Turner, T.B. & Hollander, D.H. (1957). Biology of the treponematoses based on the studies carried out at the International Treponematosis Laboratory Center of the Johns

Hopkins University under the auspices of the World Health Organization. *Monograph Series of the World Health Organization,* Vol.35, pp. 3-266, ISSN 0512-3038

Van Damme, K., Behets, F. & Ravelomanana, N. (2009). Evaluation of azithromycin resistance in *Treponema pallidum* specimens from Madagascar. *Sexually Transmitted Diseases,* Vol.36, No.12, (December 2009), pp. 775-776, ISSN 0148-5717

Walker, E.M., Howell, J.K. & You, Y. (1995). Physical map of the genome of *Treponema pallidum* subsp. *pallidum* (Nichols). *Journal of Bacteriology,* Vol.177, No.7, (April 1995), pp. 1797–1804, ISSN 0021-9193

Weinstock, G.M., Norris, S.J. & Sodergren, E. (2000). Identification of virulence genes *in silico*: infectious disease genomics, In: *Virulence mechanisms of bacterial pathogens,* Brogden, K.A., Roth, J.A., Stanton, T.B., Bolin, C.A., Minion, F.C., Wannemuehler, M.J., (Ed.), 251–261, ASM Press, ISBN 1-55581-174-4, Washington, DC, USA

Wendel, G.D., Jr, Sanchez, P.J. & Peters, M.T. (1991). Identification of *Treponema pallidum* in amniotic fluid and fetal blood from pregnancies complicated by congenital syphilis. *Obstetrics and Gynecology,* Vol.78, No.5, (November 1991), pp. 890–894, ISSN 0029-7844

Part 2

Syphilis Disease

3

History of Different Therapeutics of Venereal Disease Before the Discovery of Penicillin

Judit Forrai
Semmelweis University, Faculty of Medicine,
Institute of Public Health, Budapest
Hungary

1. Introduction

Venereal diseases are nearly as old as the history of mankind. The infections spread in exactly the same way. However, the types of diseases, our knowledge about them, and the therapies based on these have varied through the different historical periods. Nowadays we know of more than 20 types of venereal diseases, but their recognition and identification, as well as distinguishing one from the others (differential diagnosis), requires a degree of scientific knowledge that became only available as a result of the technical-scientific advances of the 20th century. Venereal diseases were known under the umbrella terms of infectious malady, pox, Venus illness, lecherous sickness and syphilis. The various names originate from the observations, scientific knowledge, and moral judgement of the given epochs.

The ancient cultures treated venereal infections as a variation of "leprosy universalis", the most widespread illness of the period. There was a reasonable amount of knowledge about how it spread and its symptoms.

The Summary of Sushruta enshrines the ancient Indian medicinal knowledge about venereal disease and its treatment. We can gain detailed information about individual illnesses, for example, about the endemic inflammation of the genitals, the stenosis of foreskin, orchiocele, or the various other chancrous changes of the genital organs. Among the recommended cures the texts mention the use of mercurial salves, a treatment known even in those early days. According to the observations, the way the "infectious malady" was transmitted could be clearly linked to the sexual act, and we can find its symptoms under the in-depth description of leprosy.

The first work summarising medicine in ancient China is the Huang-Ti Nei-Ching, *The Yellow Emperor's Classic of Internal Medicine.* In this textbook two chapters deal with venereal diseases and their treatments. Since these illnesses are transmitted through sexual intercourse and overturn the balance of the body, their treatment thus consisted of the restoration of the unity of Yin and Yang with the help of acupuncture and acupressure, along with moxa and herbs (1. picture).

From documents surviving from the period of the Egyptian Empire we know that the ancient Egyptians were excellent observers; they provided meticulous descriptions about venereal diseases and purulent discharges. The Ebers Papyrus (2. pict.) gives important formulae for the treatment of gynaecological disease, for maintaining a high level of venereal hygiene and body cult including lavage, censing, salves, the use of scents.

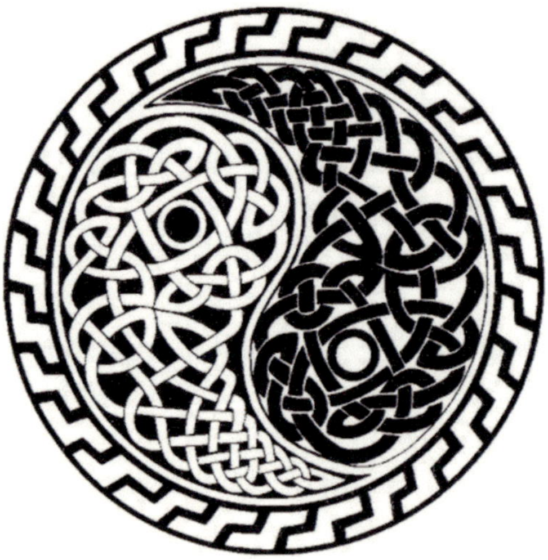

Fig. 1. Picture: Yin Yang

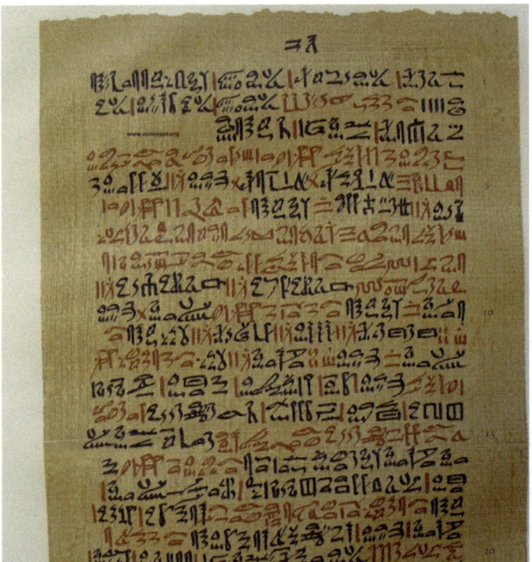

Fig. 2. Picture Ebers papyrus

Common components used for the treatment of discharges resulting from infections were garlic, acanthus resin, cow horn, the grist of vegetable seeds combined with oil, put on a sponge and placed into the vagina. In the case of men, circumcision was used to prevent venereal diseases and keep the genitals clean. In an Egyptian drawing the condom is depicted like a badge; presumably they used it as protection against venereal or tropical diseases, or maybe against flies and mosquitoes.

In the Assyrian-Babylonian culture, the Mylitta cult, in which sacred prostitution and sexuality were raised to the level of religion, put venereal diseases in the centre of attention. People tried to frighten away the "demons" with a high level of hygiene, as well as the use of herbs and amulets.

The ancient Jewish sexual practices were laid down in a religious law that became compulsory. During the Babylonian and later Egyptian Exile, relentless strictness and severe punishment were the only way to alter the customs of the neighbouring lands. Laws protected against promiscuity, prostitution, onanism, sodomy, and fornication outside marriage. The practice of circumcision and frequent bathing attest to a high level of sexual hygiene. Syphilitic infections were considered to be the retribution for fornication and the curse of Baal Peor.[1]

In Greek-Roman culture sexuality played a central role in everyday life. In 594 BC Solon founded the first state brothel, the profit of which increased the income of the city-state of Athens. Male and female sexual services existed side by side. The worship of several well-known mythological Gods and Goddesses on various holy days included placing offerings on the altar of love (Aphrodite, Venus, Dionysus, Bacchus, Phallus, Priapus, Eros, etc.)

Under the reign of Traianus (98-117 AD) the number of prostitutes in the Roman Empire exceeded 32,000. Detailed records were kept about their income and activities. Signs indicated the name of the girl working in the small cell; "occupied" and "free" notices told the patrons whether they could enter the small room filled with the smoke and scent of incense. The signboard of the brothel depicted a huge phallus.

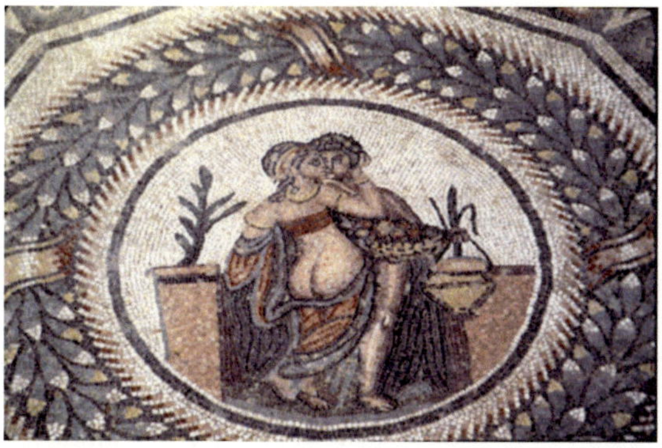

Fig. 3. Picture: 32.000 prostitute

The multi-volume works collected by Hippocrates, Galenus and Celsus mention venereal diseases and infectious maladies in several places, and clearly state their origin in the sexual act.

Women practised frequent vaginal lavage, whereas men used the contents of a small oil bottle after visiting a brothel. Pliny is a good example for one method of preventing venereal diseases. Supposedly he carried a sheep appendix or fish bladder - the predecessor of the condom - in a fold of all his togas in order to prevent infections. For Roman soldiers these aids were absolutely necessary since they were frequent visitors to the brothels - the so-called Lupanars.

---

[1] The Book of Moses, 25. 1-19

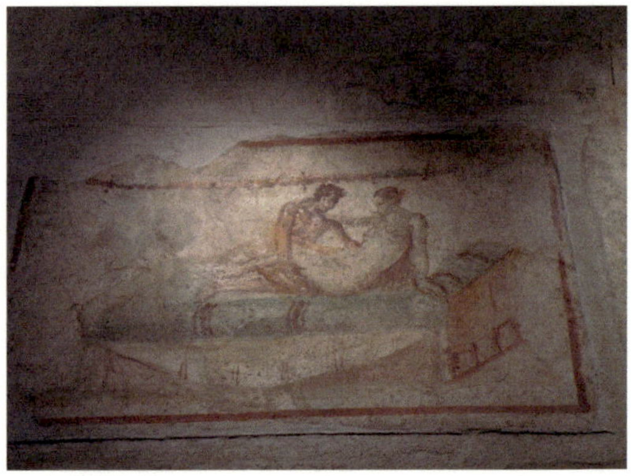

Fig. 4. Picture Lupanar in Pompei

The increasing number of brothels in Europe played an important role in the life of towns in the Middle Ages. These institutions were managed by towns, kings, princes and people holding high public offices. The prostitutes were ordered to visit on feast days and councils. When princes or nobles arrived, the inhabitants of the "house" were put at the disposal of the guests. The court of Pope Innocent IV visited Lyon between 1241 and 1251. When the court of the pope left the town, one of the cardinals said to a citizen: "*My friends, you owe us a great debt of gratitude. When we arrived in the town, we found only three brothels, and now as we leave, only one remains, but that reaches all the way from the eastern to the western gate*".

Pope Sistine IV (1478-79) built an elegant brothel.[2] Almost every town had one such establishment, which were called bordel by the French, bordello by the Italians and bordély by the Hungarians. In Hungary the first reference to brothels is about a house in Pozsony (today Bratislava, Slovakia) in 1373, which was later - in 1434 - taken into the management of the town in order to achieve greater profit. Similarly brothels were established in Eperjes (Prešov) in 1478, and in Lőcse (Levoča) and Brassó (Brašov) in 1522.

In the brothels, the hygienic laws had to be followed and cleanliness maintained in accordance with the regulations. Midwives, the proprietresses and later the town executioners were charged with the physical examination of the prostitutes, to recognize and prevent the spread of the infectious maladies.

In the 1490s Europe suffered from a deadly plague transmitted through sexual intercourse which raged in several countries. According to Lajos Nékám, a Hungarian accomplished dermatologist,[3] the emergence of diseases correspond to different eras: "Every century had its characteristic diseases, like leprosy in the 13th century, the plague in 14th century, syphilis and sudor anglicus (sweating sickness) in the 15th and 16th centuries, and these diseases had an effect on families as well as the state, just like tuberculosis and maybe cancer does nowadays."

The disease which erupted with incomparable ferocity at the end of the 15th century was considered "genius epidemicus" until the 18th century. The physicians brought up in the tradition of the Galenic school were at a loss when faced with this new epidemic and, because their master's book had no description about the disease, how it spread or ways to cure it, they were unable to help those who sought their assistance.

[2] Romea nobile admodum lupanar extruxit etiam Romana scorta is singulas hebdomadas Julium pendent Pontifici, qui census annus nonnuquam viginti milla ducatus excredit. The income of this brothel was 20,000 ducats, when a monastery paid 60 gold annually Linzbauer: Codex Sanitario Medicinalis I., II. k. 641. 1852-61, 535. Linzbauer, ibid., VI. k, 22. Linzbauer, ibid. III. lectio I. 424.

[3] Nékám, L.: From Memories of Hungarian Dermatology. Budapest, 1908. p. 54.

Since they had no other means of protection against the disease, they saw the only way of defence was the separation of the prostitutes and outsiders who were spreading it. The French king Charles VIII ordered every outsider with syphilis to leave Paris within 24 hours on pain of death in his decree published first in 1495 and again in 1498. As a result of other settlements following the lead of Paris, the roads from Besançon to Nuremberg, and from Strasbourg to Vienna became filled with persecuted and miserable wretches spreading the disease.

2. What causes this disease, where does it come from, and where did it get its name?

According to the scientists of the 16th century: Fracastorius, Fallopius, Fernelius and Girtanner[4] the causative agents were brought back to Europe by the ships of Columbus.
Others claim that in Italy and Denmark, syphilis was already raging in 1483. According to Petrus Oleus, a Danish chronicler, a contagious disease was spreading in Denmark in 1483 "which was noted under the name morbus gallicus".
Sudhoff also confirms that the disease could already be found in Europe before the time of Columbus and that it had even caused small endemics. Parrot[5], the great syphilis expert of the nineteenth century, professed the same theory. During his studies, he believed he had found syphilitic deformations on bones from French grave findings from the 11th century. It was only later that paleopathological observations confirmed the said deformations were actually caused by other diseases (osteoporosis or rachitis).
There were some who claimed that syphilis, or lues, was taken to America on Columbus's ship, and then spread among the native American Indian population that had been free from the disease until then.[6]
Another opinion held that syphilis developed as a variation of well-known tropical diseases causing raspberry-like rashes like yaws, framboesia, pian, buba, pinta, polypapilloma tropicum and Goundou, and resulting from climatic differences. Which are these diseases? Until Fritz Schaudin discovered the causative agent of syphilis in 1905, the *Treponema pallida* bacterium, it was impossible to find a cure. The "wet and dry" varieties of syphilis are in fact different members of a pathogen family that produce the same symptoms with minor

[4] Fracastorius, G.: Syphilis seu Morbuws Gallicus. Verona, 1530. exu.: Josephus Cominus, Patavii. - Fallopius G.: De morbo Gallico, posthumus 1564. - Fernel, J.: Medicamentorum facile... Francofurti 1581. Wecheleus. – C. Girtanner: Abhandlung Über die Venerische Krankheit. Gottingen, 1788.

[5] Fracastorius, G.: Syphilis seu Morbuws Gallicus. Verona, 1530. exu.: Josephus Cominus, Patavii. - Fallopius G.: De morbo Gallico, posthumus 1564. - Fernel, J.: Medicamentorum facile... Francofurti 1581. Wecheleus. – C. Girtanner: Abhandlung Über die Venerische Krankheit. Gottingen, 1788.

[6] This seems to be confirmed by the letter of Petrus Martyr written in Andalusia on April 5th 1488 to Anglerius, and written in Salamanca to Lusitanus, in which he expresses his regret that Lusitanus suffers from 'bubas' as it is called in Spanish. Torella writes that syphilis was already raging in Auvergne in the year 1493. In fact a French parliamentary decree from 1496 prescribes the relocation of sick women to designated areas, and governmental health provision. According to a priest called Delicado in 1488 syphilis was already widespread in Rapallo. From there the infection was carried to Spain, then by ship to America and from there it returned to the continent. P. M. A. Ario Lusitano, Graecas Littera Salamanticae in Pellier: Les origines la Syphilis, Toulous, Paris, 1908. Ruy Diaz de Isla in Bloch: Der Ursprung der Syphilis, Jena, 1901. Torella, G.: Tractus, cum consiliis contra morbum gallicum cui adjicitur in fine, Rome, 1497.

variations due to the climate. According to recent genetic research[7] syphilis, which terrorised Europe for almost five centuries, was imported from the Americas by the crew of Christopher Columbus, who presumably carried the pathogen on their skins instead of sexually. A molecular genetic family tree analysis of the disease by US researchers has shown that Treponema pallida, the infectious agent causing syphilis (lues), is most closely related to Treponema pertenue which is responsible for a serious tropical skin disease called framboesia. Researcher Kristin Harper says, "*Some people think it is a really ancient disease that our earliest human ancestors would have had. Other people think it came from the New World. What we found is that syphilis or a progenitor came from the New World to the Old World and this happened pretty recently in human history,*" she added[8].

Researchers in Chicago examined numerous bone remains from both the Old and the New World as the presence of syphilis is attested by breaks in the bones so characteristic of it. Harper's group examined the evolution of the pathogens: they scrutinized the evolutionary links of 26 strains of the Treponema bacteria, including two Spirochaeta species never examined before genetically that cause framboesia in some remote areas of Guyana and South America. Genetic data showed framboesia to be an ancient disease while syphilis, spread through sexual contact, proved to be relatively recent. However, of all tropical species, this is the only one that remains active in the cooler climate of Europe. This is an important step forward in the evolution of the species - however, the way this occurred remains obscure.

There is credible genetic evidence that the syphilis which terrorized Europe for nearly five centuries was "imported" by Christopher Columbus's sailors returning from America. However, the virus probably travelled on the skin of the sailors and not in a venereal way. American genetic family-tree research proved that the nearest "cousin" of the lues pathogen (the Treponema pallida bacterium) is the serious tropical skin disease framboesia which is caused by Treponema pertenue. According to the researcher Kristin Harper, "Some people think it is a really ancient disease that our earliest human ancestors would have had. Other people think it came from the New World. What we found is that syphilis or a progenitor came from the New World to the Old World and this happened pretty recently in human history," she added.

Still others say that the disease arrived from eastern India, Persia and the Far East. This claim was supported by the research of Adachi[9] who believed he had found the signs of syphilis on bones from the Neolithic Age in Japan. The scientific analysis of pre-Columbian discoveries on the American continent came into the focus of attention at the end of the nineteenth century. The scientists believed that, if they were unable to find syphilitic deformations on the bones, then Columbus's soldiers could not have been infected with the disease. Farquhason (1875), Jones (1876), Morgan (1892), Ashmead (1895), Moore (1897), Lamb (1898), etc. confirmed the pre-Columbian existence of syphilis when they announced

[7] Harper KN, Liu H, Ocampo PS, Steiner BM, Martin A, Levert K, Wang D, Sutton M, Armelagos GJ.: The sequence of the acidic repeat protein (arp) gene differentiates venereal from nonvenereal Treponema pallidum subspecies, and the gene has evolved under strong positive selection in the subspecies that causes syphilis. FEMS Immunol Med Microbiol. 2008 Aug; 53(3):322-32. Epub 28 June 2008

[8] Kristin Harper: On the Origins of Syphilis. PLoS Neglected Tropical Diseases. 16 January 2008

[9] Adachi, B.: Syphilis in der Steinzeit in Japan. Arch. Dermat. u. Syphilis 54. 1. 1901. Regöly-Gy. Mérei: Systematic pathology of the palaeonthropic and later remains, Budapest, 1962.

their findings. Recent immunological research[10] also confirms that the disease arrived in America from Mongolia through the Bering Strait nearly 40,000 years ago.
From all of these facts it can be concluded that we have no exact knowledge about the origin of syphilis.
This cruel epidemic broke out in different countries at the same time in the 16th century - with deadly consequences. In the early period those who diagnosed it and distinguished it from other already known diseases gave it new names, usually after different regions or countries. It is quite probable that the names reflect the course of the disease, which means that the route of the pandemic can be followed in this way.
Sibbens *in Scotland* (Button Scurvy); Radesynge (rada- bad, synge epidemic) *in Sweden and Norway;* Juttlandian disease *in Juttland;* Dittmarsian or Holsteinian disease *in Holstein. In Spain*: La bubas, Postillas, Curiale (court disease), Patursa passio turpis Saturnia; *in France*: Grosse verole, La gorre Morbus Neapolizanus, Scor, Scorra; *in England:* Grandor, Mala Franzos, Morbus Burdigalensis; *in Germany:* Böse Kratze, Mala Franzos; in *Italy*: La Clavela, Morbus Galli. But other associations also played a part in the naming process. (5. picture)

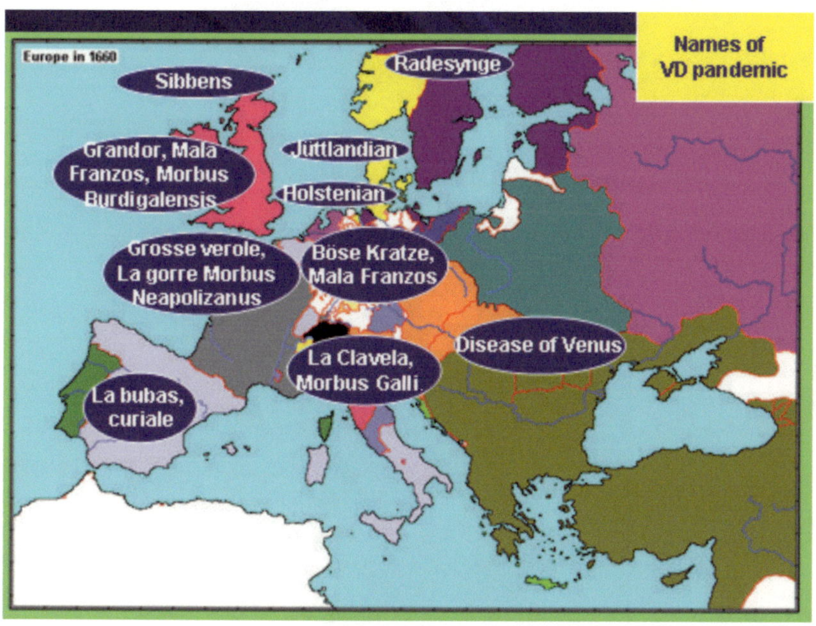

Fig. 5. Picture Names of Europian VD epidemic

In the 16th century Fernelius, a Parisian teacher (6. picture), called it lues, while the Italian Fracastorius (7. picture)named it syphilis. Fracastorius[11] took the name from the Greek mythology. We can read about syphilis in the Iliad (XXIV. 585-621). Niobe (a daughter of Tantalus) had seven sons and seven daughters. The name of one of the sons was Sipylus, which is identical with the name of the city founded by his grandfather and the mountain standing nearby. Niobe was so proud of her children that she demanded the Gods worship

[10] Ruffié J., Sournia, Ch.: Die Seuchen in der Geschichte der Menschheit, Stuttgart, 1987. Klett-Cotta.
[11] Mythological Encyclopaedia I.II. ed.: Sz. A. Tokarev. Gondolat. Budapest, 1988.

her above Apollo and Artemis, the children of Leto. The two children of Leto shot all fourteen children with arrows to avenge their humiliation. The Gods were moved by the pain of Niobe, and they brought her and her children to Mount Sipylus and turned them to stone.

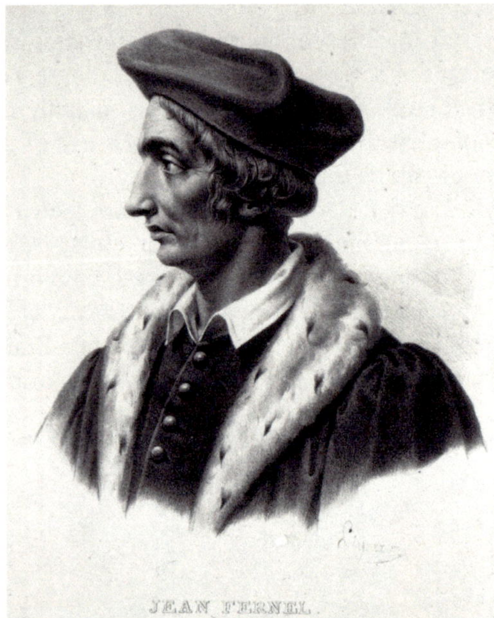

Fig. 6. Picture Jean Fernelius

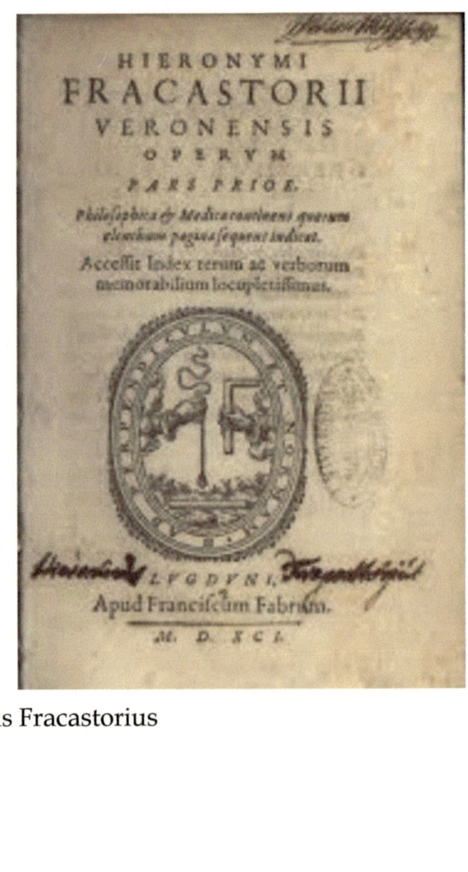
HIERONYMI
FRACASTORII
VERONENSIS
OPERVM
PARS PRIOR.
Philosophica & Medica continens: quorum elenchum pagina sequens indicat.
Accessit Index rerum ac verborum memorabilium locupletissimus.
LVGDVNI,
Apud Franciscum Fabrum.
M. D. XCI.

Fig. 7. Picture Hieronimus Fracastorius

Fracastorius changes this tale to the following: Syphilus, the shepherd of King Alchitous, suffering from the rays of the sun, curses the Gods and says that their flock cannot rival that of Alchitous in either beauty or in size, and thus the king deserves to be worshipped as a God. Apollo observes as the shepherd builds an altar to the new God. In his rage, he curses the shepherd with a hideous, gluey, infectious disease that is called syphilis after its first victim.

The Greek expression 'siflos' means empty, in vain, formless, cripple, disease, incomplete in a figurative sense, handicapped, or shameful. According to another etymological explanation it is a compound consisting of the words 'sys': pig and 'filia': friendship, meaning that the disease originates from an unclean, infectious love. Still another explanation states that Fracastorius coined it from the Arabic words Sifl or Sufl, which mean below, inferior and which could refer to the place or manner of the infection.

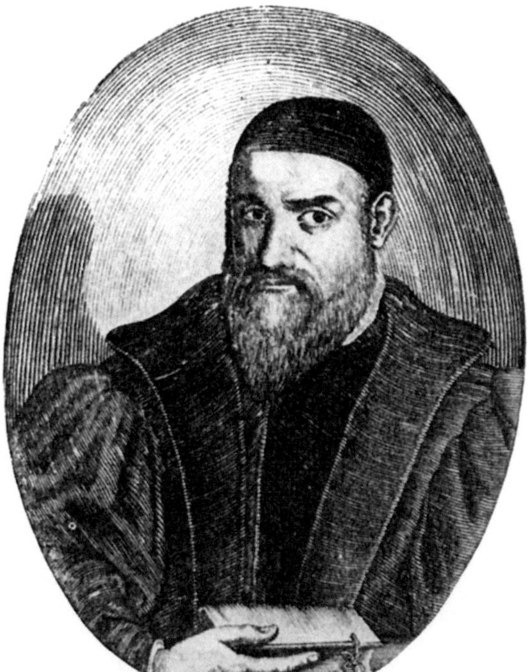

Fig. 8. Picture Girolamo Fallopius

The epidemic expansion of the disease took its toll among all classes and both sexes. Even royalty had its own interest in fighting it. The "great" kings Charles VIII and Francis I of France, Holy Roman Emperor Maximillian I, Pope Alexander VI (Borgia) and his whole family, Tamás Bakócz (1442-1521) Hungarian cardinal and heir apparent to the papal throne, and George IV of England all suffered and died of lues.

Due to the similarity to the medieval disease leprosy, in the beginning the therapy consisted of the same remedies such as sulphuric water, violet oil, minium. Later, based on the Eastern example, they used mercury for the first time as a remedy for syphilis in Europe.

Fallopius (8. picture) (1523-1562) in his work titled Sive Morbus Gallicus discusses the results of 5-8 autopsies conducted during a single year, the subjects of which all died from the Gallic disease. He was curiously investigating the causes of the deformations and was surprised to observe that the "solution continui", which was present in almost every organ in the body of a syphilis victim, spared only the liver. The first written report about a modern condom originates from Fallopius who, in 1564, attributed great importance to the apparatus made from a small piece of linen in the fight against syphilis. He states (De Morbo Gallico) that he conducted his experiment with 1100 people who thanks to the condom avoided infection with the illness which in that period usually led to death in a very short time.

However, he frankly admits in his recommendation that the disease cannot be defeated. Therefore, according to the fashion of the time, he recommends the use of guaiac tree and Sarsaparilla.[12]

The guaiac (9. picture)is a holy tree (Guaiacum officinale, lignum sanctum) which arrived in Europe around 1508 from the torrid zone of America: South Florida, Bahamas, Cuba, San Domingo. In 1578 Péter Mélius wrote a detailed report[13] about de Ligni guaiaco also known as French tree and guaiac tree. Its active constituents can be found in its resin which has an acrid taste and consists of resin, volatile oil, guaiaguttin, rubber, vanillin and saponin. It has a diaphoretic and laxative effect. Its use was recommended by several other authorities, including Ulrich von Hutten who wrote a separate paper about this excellent drug.

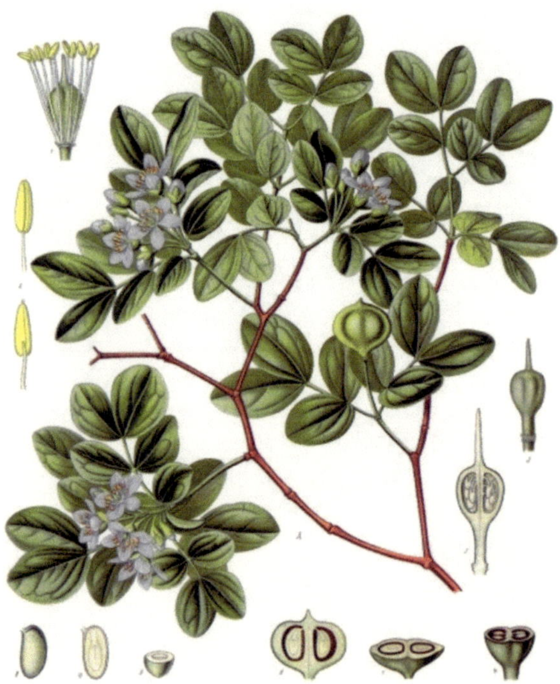

Fig. 9. Picture Guaiac tree

[12] "Quauis similicia ista diuersa habeant partes, tamen Sarsaparilia, Guaiacum, argentum vivuum uniformia sunt."

[13] P. Melius: 1578 Herbárium About the uses, names and growths of trees and grasses 1578. Kolozsvár, repr. Bukarest, 1979

Another important element of the fight against syphilis was the herbal decoction of sarsaparilla (10. picture), a plant with American origins. Its name came from the Mexican sarsaparilla, China root. They used it for its blood cleansing and appetizer properties. In a high dose it causes diarrhoea, salivary secretion, perspiration and a high urinary output. Therefore, in accordance with the ideas of the period, it was an excellent means of purging the body.

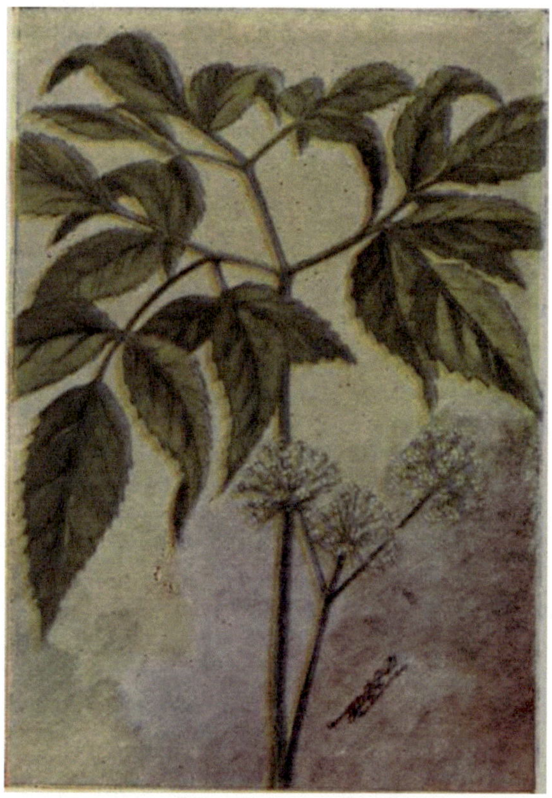

Fig. 10. Ábra Sarsaparilla

The third important herb, Sassafras (11. picture), is also of American origin and has been known in Europe only since the 16th century. Sassafras officinalis, which belongs to the Lauraceae family, is endemic to Canada. Its root, wood and bark are each used as medicine. According to Wittstein the origin of the word goes back to "sal safras" meaning shattered stone. Its active constituent can be found in the volatile oil. Its effects are also diaphoretic and increase the metabolism. Sassafras was first described in 1574 by Nicolaus Monardes, a Sevillian physician.[14]

Since the origin of syphilis was believed to be strongly connected with the discovery of America, it was only natural to assume that the cure for the disease could also be accomplished by using drugs and herbs from the New World. The herbs used had a purging effect, causing perspiration, diarrhoea and a high urinal output. The theory was that

[14] Kazay E.: Apothecary Lexicon. Nagybánya, 1900.

consuming a high dose of these herbs would result in the purging of the body and "cleansing" of the blood. Beside the use of American cures in Europe, one of the most important economic considerations was the dramatic increase in drugs imported - a major part of commerce - as had already been mentioned by Paracelsus. According to him, there was a linear connection between the guaiac cure and the profit making aspirations of Fugger House (12. picture).[15]

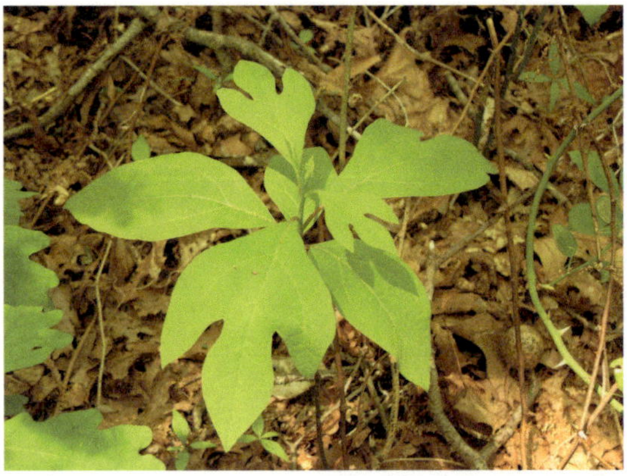

Fig. 11. Picture Sassafras

Finally we have to consider the psychological factors as well. The patients were willing do anything in order to be cured - even to make huge financial sacrifices, especially where a new and expensive medicine from another continent was concerned. However, despite these excellent remedies, the fury of syphilis did not show any sign of weakening. The herbs imported from America were not as effective as they had first seemed.

The Eastern cure, mercury, was used carefully since they considered it a potent poison based on Greek and Roman tradition. According to Aristotle it can kill a rat in even a very small dose. Pliny[16] stated that it corrodes everything except gold, and therefore recommended that it was not to be used internally, only externally as a salve. The salve cure was based on lard, cock's fat, butter, oil, turpentine or the saliva of a hungry man. Its active constituent was quicksilver which, when combined with the base, loses its fluidity, "undergoes mortification", and disintegrates into smaller parts which enables it to enter the body more easily.

The deadly disease was also affecting the Turkish sailors. Barbarossa, the admiral of Suleiman I's (12. picture)navy and also king of Algiers, was the first to give a mercurial pill to his infected soldiers, and the medicine was later named after him. This so-called Barbarossa pill turned out to be effective. The court physician of Francis I also mentions its good effects. The Barbarossa pill contained mercury combined with perfume essence and fruit flour, and then doused in lemon juice. The recipe, once thought long lost, can be found in the book of Astruc published in 1788.[17] This means that the merit of the first mercuric medicine administered through the mouth (internally) belongs to Arabic medicine and not to Paracelsus.

---

[15] Paracelsus: Paragranum. Gyomaendrőd, 1989. Helikon, p. 111.

[16] Plinius sec. Historiae Naturalis Libri XXXIII., XXXII., Biponti 1984., p. 2000

[17] Astruc, J.: De morbis veneris Libri sex. Paris, 1788. Guillelmun Cavelier 167. p.

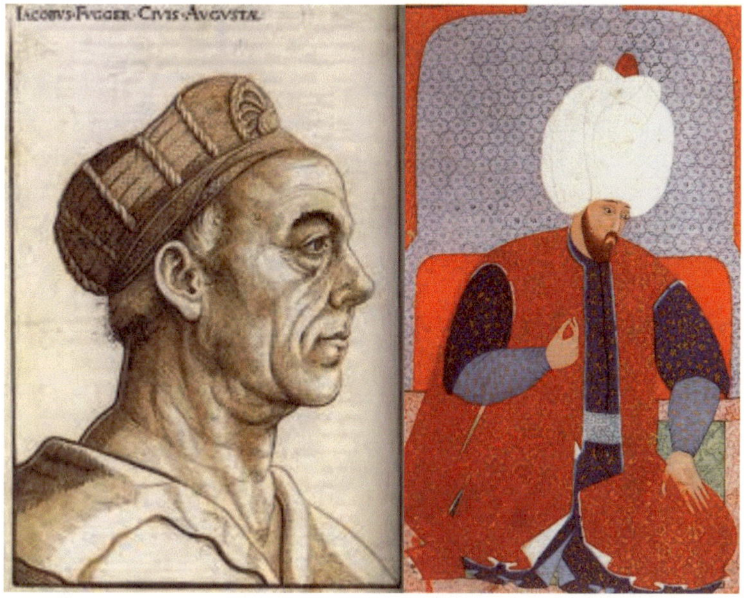

Fig. 12. Picture Fugger and Suleiman I.

The identification of the disease is not unambiguous. Fallopius speaks about gonorrhoea gallica, that is gonorrhoea caused by syphilis, while Fernelius believes that urethral discharge (a symptom of gonorrhoea) is a form of syphilis. Clearly they merge the two diseases, and that is how the basis of theory of unity developed.

In the 17th century one of the eminent figures of the iatrochemical school, Étienne Blanchard,[18] wrote a summary work about the treatment of syphilis. According to his ideas, which were based on chemical principles, syphilis emerges from the combination of certain acids and blood. He calls this phenomenon acrimony. The primary cause of the infection is the coitus act with an unclean person. The infection enters the healthy blood from the infected blood through the genital organs. The other method of infection is breast-feeding, through the nipples. Therefore the disease spreads not causa epidemica, but from one person to the other (causa particulary et singulary).

Since the origin of the disease was explained based on the iatrochemical school, it seems understandable that the combination of the blood and the infection creates another discharge, compound, an acidic or alkaline acrimony, and therefore the aim of the cure is to neutralize these substances. The process of the cure: first the bowels have to be cleared with medicaments consisting of Venetian turpentine, extractum rhei, cremo tartan, extr. catholoco, mercurius dulcis, mercurius preacipatus albus. After that, diuretics are used (Alkanna root, tea, Peruvian balm, myrrh). This is followed by purging (decoctions, drops and pills) and later by antacid and tempering medicines: China root, Sarsaparilla, Sassafras, mastic, coral, etc.)

Strong emphasis is placed on the washing of the body, and fluid intake: the consumption of sweet milk, tea and coffee. Drinking wine and smoking is prohibited. There are different procedures for sweating. The patient has to be seated on a stool, a rug placed beneath his

[18] Etienne Blanchard: Traite de la Verole. Paris, 1688.

feet, his whole body covered by blankets like a tent. Then a heat source has to be set in front of the stool inside the blankets. A hot brick can also be used as a heat source. According to the ideas of the period, the use of surgical plasters was also recommended.
The use of condoms (13. picture) was one of the means for the defence against the disease. In the case of this important and handy aid, again both the name and origin can vary quite dramatically; it is known as fireman's syringe, rubbers, Port Said Garter and Venus glove. The English call it French letter, the French Capote Anglaise (English hood). However, most commonly it is referred to as condom.

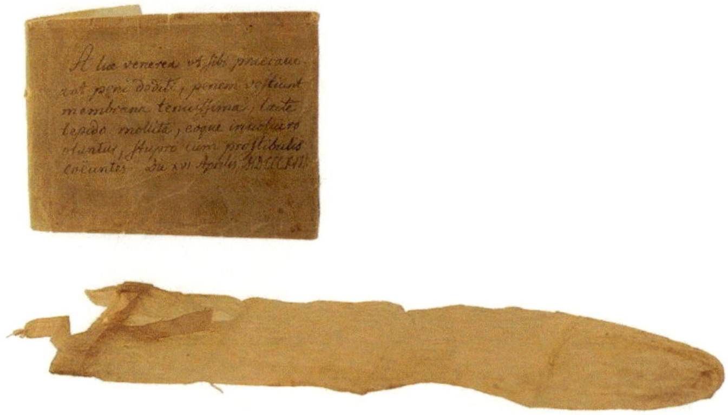

Fig. 13. Ábra Fracastorius, condom

According to some sources this name comes from the Latin word 'condere', meaning 'protect'; others trace it back to the idiom Cum Domino. There are others who claim it got its name from the French town of Condom. According to some the physician of Charles II (Stuart), Quondom, offered the "assurance cap" to his king, in order to help decide the question of inheritance and prevent the birth of illegitimate offspring. Another version states that a colonel by this name serving in Cromwell's army ordered his soldiers to use this important protection. The remains of five condoms were found in a bottle during excavations in the castle.
According to contemporary records, the Venus glove was already known in Paris by 1655. In a letter written by Madame de Sévigné to her daughter in 1671, she refers to it as the 'French glove' and recommends its use in order to avoid that certain danger. Marquis De Sade and Casanova (14. picture) used it not only as a contraceptive, but also against the spreading of venereal diseases. According to the advice of Casanova, the best way to ensure the condom is without fault is to inflate it before use.
In 1701 there was already a shop selling condoms in England. Information about the product was recorded and circulated in the form of poems:

To protect you from fear and shame
there are no faulty ones here to blame
Don't let your Venus passion be quenched.
Do as nature bids you and shield your health.

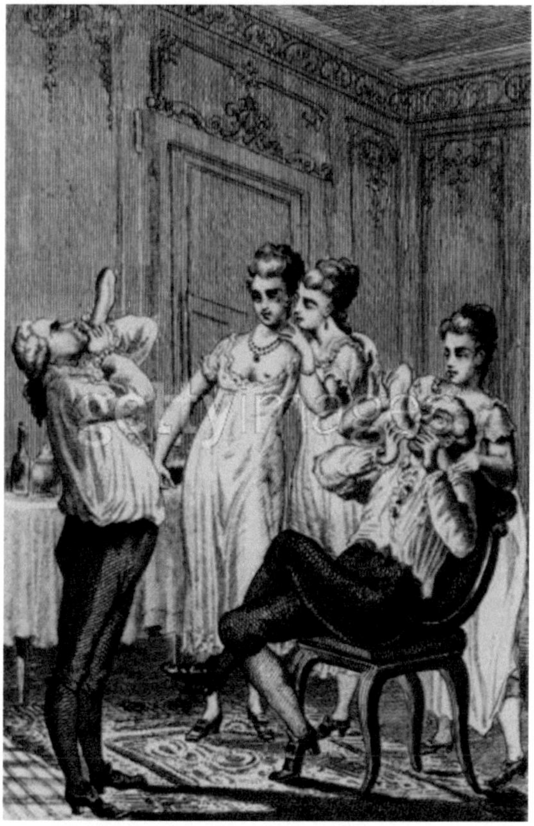

Fig. 14. Ábra Casanova and condom test

Mrs Philips and Mrs Perkins's factory became the biggest condom supplier of London in the 18th century. They manufactured for the wholesale market, as well as for envoys, foreigners, lords and ship captains. Orders came from Spain, Italy and, of course, France. However, just as in the case of other new and profitable businesses, this one too had its opponents who tried to scientifically prove that this special "assurance cap" was popular not for the protection it provided against infection but for what it represented, namely prostitution and immorality. With this they defined and stigmatised it for centuries to come: the place of the condom in a hypocritic world.

In medical circles the hesitation towards the condom was caused by the lack of evidence for its effectiveness on the one hand, and the unrestrained sexuality and the inability to check marital fidelity they said it enabled on the other. Most of the records mention the condom as an object of prostitution that the prostitutes themselves sold.

Naturally the notions about venereal diseases defined the way they were cured. Venereal disease, which was regarded as a single disease for centuries after the medieval pandemic of syphilis, actually covered many different illnesses. This caused a plethora of misunderstandings and mistakes in the identification, isolation and treatment of venereal infections.

The isolation of three venereal diseases, chancroid, gonorrhoea and syphilis, was achieved only in the 19th century. Cockurne (1715) was the first to treat syphilis and gonorrhoeal discharge as separate diseases. Later Balfour, Ellis and Tode vigorously denied that these diseases were the same, until the failed experiment of John Hunter (1728-1793) (15. picture). As is well known, he injected the gonorrhoeal discharge of a patient into the foreskin of a healthy person. Unfortunately, however, Hunter did not know that the patient had syphilis as well as gonorrhoea. That is why the experiment, which clearly proved that syphilis emerges from gonorrhoea, set back the differential diagnosis of these two diseases for many decades.

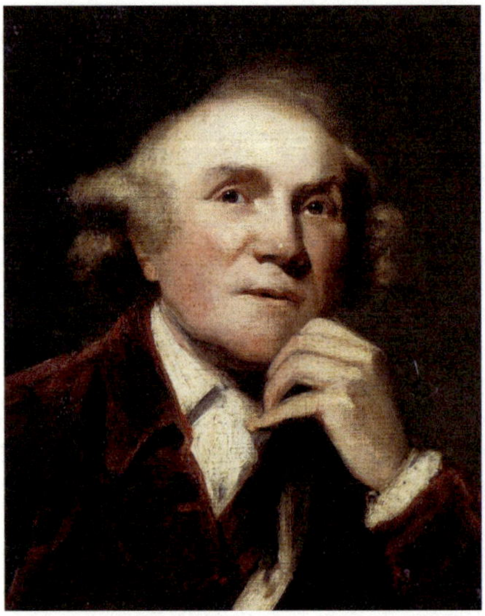

Fig. 15. Picture John Hunter

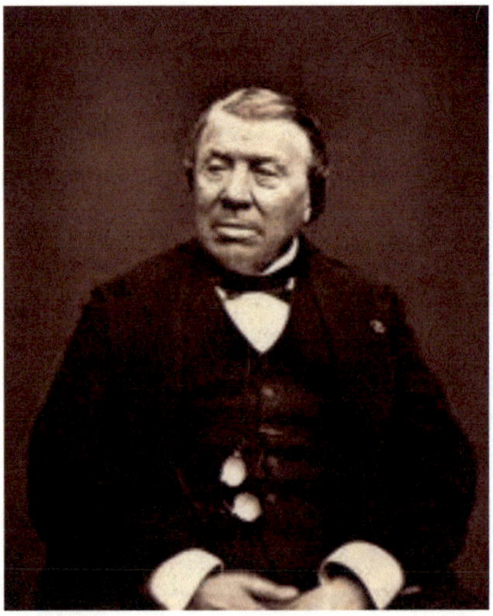

Fig. 16. Picture Philippe Record

As we have seen, the theory of uniformity dominated perceptions about venereal diseases until Bell (1793), Frank (1797) and Hernandez (1812) tried to prove that the two diseases

differ from one another. In 1831 Ricord (16. picture) conducted more than 667 gonorrhoeal and 1500 syphilitic inoculations, which clearly confirmed the fact that gonorrhoea can only emerge from a gonorrhoeal infection, and syphilis from a syphilitic infection. Based on Ricord, syphilis was separated into three stages: primary, second ulcerous stage, and the final so-called late state.
Concerning the treatment, physicians were divided into two groups. One group argued for mercury treatment, the other for non-mercurial therapies. Mercury poisoning occurring as a result of the uncertain amount of administered mercury made the condition of the patient deteriorate even further in addition to the uncured or recurring syphilis. According to Poór's statistical records, 60% of the patients treated with mercury returned with recurring syphilis and additional mercury poisoning. Therefore the iodine[19] recommended by Wallace (1835) was applied in the form of mineral water. Its harmlessness was regarded as its greatest advantage and use since, in contrast to mercury iodine, it is not poisonous. Gonorrhoea, also known as the clap, is an infectious disease localized on the mucous membranes; its causative agent was discovered by Neisser (17. picture) in 1879.

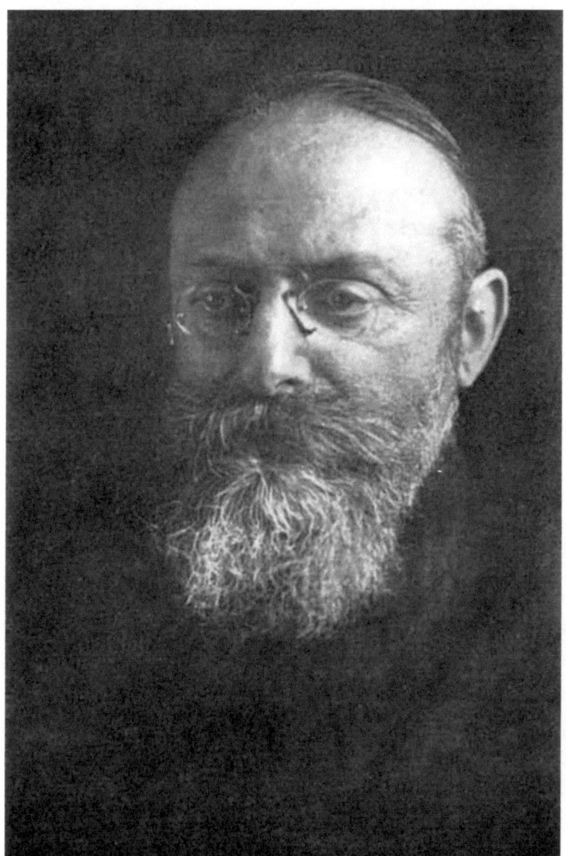

Fig. 17. Picture Albert Ludwig Sigesmund Neisser

[19] Melly-Doros: The issue of venereal diseases in Budapest. Budapest, 1930. p. 27.

The Gram-negative Neisseria gonorrhoae bacterium was named after him. In fact, gonorrhoea was considered the most widespread infectious venereal disease at the beginning of the 20th century. According to contemporaneous German statistics 80-100% of the men suffered from this disease. Our only information about the number of infected women comes from the women arrested during police raids (80% suffered from syphilis). Ricord stated the following concerning the complications of the purulent infections: "When gonorrhoea starts only God knows when it is going to end."[20] It can result in urethral, prostatic inflammation epididymitis, and even infertility in women. In its later stages it can cause arthritis through the bloodstream, and eye infection during childbirth.

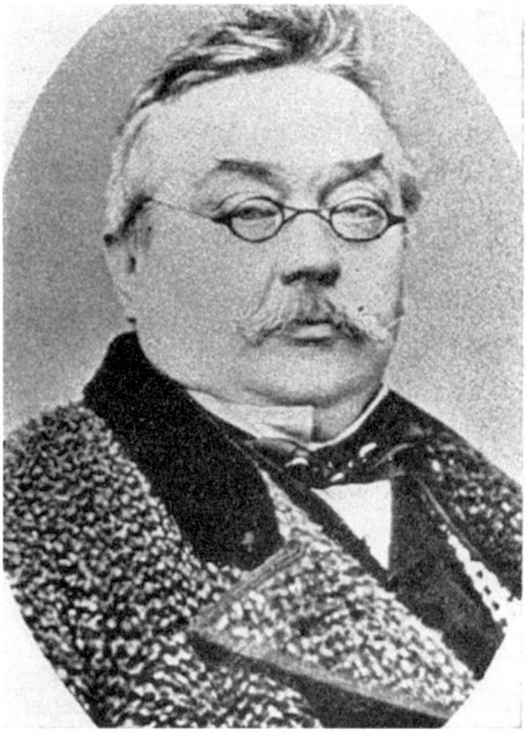

Fig. 18. Picture Ferdinand von Hebra

The experiment series which proved that syphilis and gonorrhoea are different diseases did not change the attitude of physicians in one fell swoop, since it was still impossible to separate chancroid and syphilis from one another.[21] That is how the two sides emerged: the side of the theory of unity, according to whom chancroid and syphilis were in fact the same disease. Representatives included Ricord, Zeissl, Sigmund, Kaposi, Auspitz and Schwimmer. And the side proclaiming duality considering them to be two separate diseases. Representatives included Bassereau, Laroyenne, Fournier, Diday, Mauriac, and Poór.[22]

[20] Ivan Bloch: The sexual life of our period. Budapest. Dante. 1907. p. 334.

[21] Sámuel Róna: The sexual or venereal diseases. Budapest. Hungarian Medical Book Publication Group. 1893.

[22] Melly-Doros: The issue of venereal diseases in Budapest. Budapest, 1930. p.27.

Hebra (18. picture) and Sigmund were excellent dermatologists at the second medical school in Vienna. At the University of Vienna patients were treated according to the best knowledge of the period. The syphilis ward of the General State Hospital had been providing care since 1869.[23] It offered diet, body hygiene, bathing, injection and irrigational therapies, as well as cures using patches and bandages. Of course, they also recommended washes, dusting powders, medicine injections, anointments, inhalation treatments, censing and the use of suppositories in order to cure syphilis.[24]
The embrocating procedure on five areas of the body was regarded as a new treatment: on the shins, thighs, chest, stomach and upper arm.[25] The evening was considered the best time for the treatment; these time recommendations are suggestive of traditional medicine. In Pest-Buda Poór was the first docent habilitated in dermatology and syphiligraphy in 1858-59. He studied the field in Vienna, and later worked in the dermatology ward[26] of the St Rókus hospital, where half of the patient suffered from syphilis.[27] Poór worked on syphilisation. Using experiments based on the Jenner's vaccination technique physicians all over Europe tried to discover a vaccine against syphilis. The vaccination experiments failed everywhere however, not just in Paris.[28]

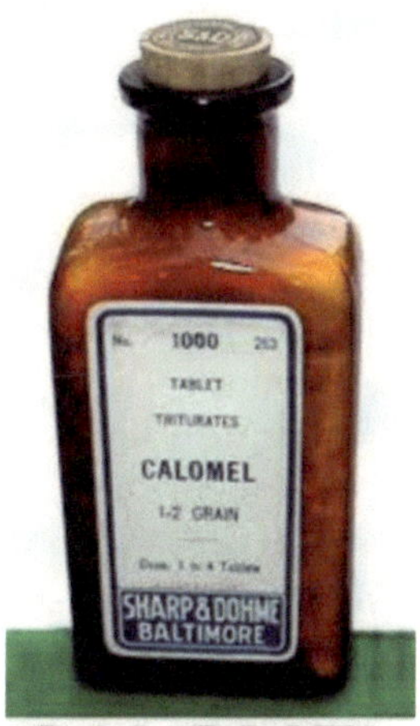

CALOMEL

Fig. 19. Picture Calomel

In order to avoid the toxic effect of mercury, they found that the injection beneath the skin of the patient was the only method which could avoid the symptoms of poisoning caused by the high dose of mercury. **Sublimate** was used by Hunter and Hebra for the first time in an amount of 25 (SMER); it did not cause any salivation. The other treatment called **Calomel**

[23] Sigmund K. Receipt samples from the infirmary of the University of Vienna. Pest. Heckenast. 1871. p. 3.
[24] Ibid. pp. 4 -15.
[25] Sigmund K.: The embrocation treatment for the cure of syphilis types. The book press of the Hungarian Royal University. 1868. p. 12.
[26] Schwimmer E.: The actual state of the treatments of syphilis. Khor and Wien. 1880. p. 3, 7.
[27] I. Poór: Iodine, the sure and harmless cure of syphilis. Gyógyászat. 37. 9 Sept 1888. p. 435.
[28] I. Poór: The value of the Bujaev-vaccination (syphidisatio) concerning the cure of syphilis. Gyógyászat. 34. 29 Aug. 1858. 560.p.

(19. picture) was first used used by Scarenzi; it often caused abscess at the point of injection, and salivation could also occur.[29]

The other docent in Budapest dealing with syphilis was Ernő Schwimmer who habilitated in 1871. Since there was no dermatology ward, he was appointed physician of the virulent exanthema ward of the barrack hospital in 1857. He was the first to use antiseptics for the treatment of variolar processes. He established a dermatology and syphidology ward and department in Kolozsvár (today Cluj Napoca, Romania) in 1874, the first in Hungary. In 1880 Schwimmer, who had already received the title of professor extraordinary, gained permission to move his public dispensary from the polyclinic to the clinic. In 1885 he established a dermatology and syphilis ward with 130 beds in the St Stephen hospital. Finally the dermatology and syphidology department was established in 1892, headed by Schwimmer.

His treatment procedure clearly shows - similarly to all the contemporaneous treatments - a wide scale of possible but unsuccessful cures. These treatments were the following:

1. Mercury treatment
   a. internal mercury treatment with the help of different pills, Dzsoni, Hufeland, Dupuytren, Mauriac, etc., van Swieten, Sigmund types. Calomel, iodine mercury preparations e.g. the Ricord type,
   b. external mercury treatment in the form of: 1. censing, 2. bath, 3 embrocation, 4. injection beneath the skin
2. Iodine treatment with different iodine preparations in the form of: potassium iodine, sodium iodine, fermium iodine and iodoform
3. The use of herbs in the form of decoctions: sassafras, guaiac tree, sarsaparilla, burdock root, China bark, e.g. Zittman type decoction, other herbs like tayuya, pilocarpin, etc.
4. Various minerals: gold, silver, platinum
5. Water cure: warm water - thermal springs containing sulphur and iodine; cold water - the Priessnitz methods
6. Various other methods: - syphidisation (vaccination) / failed experiments - dietetics

The last quarter of the 19th century was the period of great discoveries in experimental medicine. The development of the chemical industry, experiments with dyes and compounds, and bacterial discoveries all opened new avenues to cure infectious diseases. In 1905 Schaudin and Hoffman discovered the causative agent of syphilis, Treponema pallida, Wasserman composed the method which was named after him that made it possible to detect the disease in blood plasma. The new serum diagnostics made the explicit identification of the disease possible.[30] This method meant that not only the already infected patients could be diagnosed but the latent cases as well.

The new dyeing methods created the base for chemotherapy. They tried to treat malaria cases with methylene blue, and later tried malaria remedies on lues patients in accordance with the fashionable ideas of the period. In the Kolozsvár dermatology clinic patients were treated with atoxyl. In 1909 Ehrlich, with Hata's help, discovered Salvarsan after 606 experiments.

The domestic and international response to the effective, pinpoint accurate "magical balls" was unambiguous. Unfortunately it later transpired that Salvarsan (20. picture) needed to

---

29 Schwimmer E.: The actual state of the treatments of syphilis. Khor and Wien. 1880. p. 3, 7.

30 Marschalkó T.: Weekly Medical . 1909. p. 788.

be improved, and the new type was placed on market under the name Neosalvarsan. A regulation provided for the use of Salvarsan in hospitals to be financed by the national treasury, meaning that the state bore the costs of the treatment. It was penicillin, discovered by Fleming in 1942, that finally provided the solution to syphilis which had existed for so many decades.

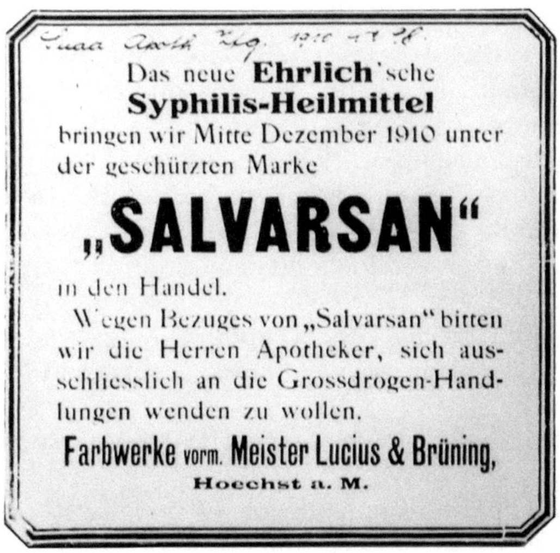
Das neue Ehrlich'sche
Syphilis-Heilmittel
bringen wir Mitte Dezember 1910 unter
der geschützten Marke
„SALVARSAN“
in den Handel.
Wegen Bezuges von „Salvarsan“ bitten
wir die Herren Apotheker, sich aus-
schliesslich an die Grossdrogen-Hand-
lungen wenden zu wollen.
Farbwerke vorm. Meister Lucius & Brüning,
Hoechst a. M.

Fig. 20. Picture Salvarsan

3. References

Adachi, B.: Syphilis in der Steinzeit in Japan. Arch. Dermat. u. Syphilis 54. 1. 1901. Regöly-Mérei, Gy. : Systematic pathology of the palaeonthropic and later remains , Budapest, 1962.

Astruc, J.: De morbis veneris Libri sex. Paris, 1788. Guillelmun Cavelier p. 167.

Bloch, I.: The sexual life of our period. Budapest. Dante. 1907. p. 334.

Blankard, É.: Traite de la Verole, Paris. 1688.

Fallopius, G.: De morbo Gallico VEnetiis 1574. Neapolitani.

Fracastorius, G.: Syphilis seu Morbuws Gallicus. Verona, 1530. exu.: Josephus Cominus, Patavii. - Fallopius G.: De morbo Gallico, posthumus 1564. - Fernel, J.: Medicamentorum facile... Francofurti 1581. Wecheleus. - C. Girtanner: Abhandlung Über die Venerische Krankheit. Gottingen, 1788.

Harper, K.: On the Origins of Syphilis. PLoS Neglected Tropical Diseases. 16 January 2008

Harper KN, Liu H, Ocampo PS, Steiner BM, Martin A, Levert K, Wang D, Sutton M, Armelagos GJ.: The sequence of the acidic repeat protein (arp) gene differentiates venereal from nonvenereal Treponema pallidum subspecies, and the gene has evolved under strong positive selection in the subspecies that causes syphilis. FEMS Immunol Med Microbiol. 2008 Aug;53 (3):322-32. Epub 28 June 2008

Isla, Ruy Diaz de: in Bloch: Der Ursprung der Syphilis, Jena, 1901. Torella, G.: Tractus, cum consiliis contra morbum gallicum cui adjicitur in fine, Rome, 1497.

Kazay E.: Apothecary Lexicon. Nagybánya, 1900.

Linzbauer X.: Codex Sanitario Medicinalis I., II. k. 641. 1852-61, 535., VI. k, 22., III. lectio I. 424.
Lusitano, P. M. A. Gr. Littera Salamanticae in Pellier: Les origines la Syphilis, Toulous, Paris 1908.
Marschalkó T.:Weekly Medical . 1909. 788.p.
Melius, P.: About the uses, names and growts of trees and grases 1578. Kolosvarott, repr. Bukarest, 1979
Melly-Doros: The issue of venereal diseases in Budapest. Budapest, 1930. p. 27.
Mythological Encyclopaedia I.II. ed.: Sz.A. Tokarev. Gondolat. Budapest, 1988.
Nékám, L.: From the memories of Hungarian Dermatology. Budapest, 1908. 54.
Paracelsus: Paragranum. Gyomaendrőd, 1989. Helikon, p. 111.
Parrot, J.: Les travaux relatifs a l'histoire de la Syphilis. Rev. Sci, 1882.
Plinius sec. Historiae Naturalis Libri XXXIII., XXXII., Biponti 1984., p. 2000.
Poór,I.: The value of the Bujaev-vaccination(syphilisatio) concerning the cure of syphilis. Gyógyászat. 34. 1858. aug. 29. p. 560.
Póór, I.: Iodine, the sure and harmless cure of syphilis. Gyógyászat. 37. 1888. szept. 9. p. 435.
Róna S: The sexual or venereal diseases. Budapest. Hungarian Medical Book Publication Group. 1893. p. 15.
Ruffié J., Sournia, Ch.: Die Seuchen in der Geschichte der Menschheit, Stuttgart, 1987. Klett-Cotta.
Schwimmer E.: The actual state of the treatments of syphilis. Khor and Wien. 1880. p. 3. 7. Sigmund K. Receipt samples from the infirmary of the University of Vienna. Pest. Heckenast. 1871. p. 3.
Sigmund K.: The embrocation treatment for the cure of syphilis types. The book-press of the Hungarian Royal University. 1868. p. 12.

4

Psychiatric Manifestations of Neurosyphilis

Fabian Friedrich and Martin Aigner
Department of Psychiatry and Psychotherapy,
Division of Social Psychiatry,
Medical University of Vienna
Austria

1. Introduction

1.1 Historical aspects

The first case of syphilis occurred in Europe around the year 1493. Martin Alonzo Pinzon, commander of one of the three ships of Christopher Columbus, is considered as first documented victim of syphilis. The term "syphilis" was first described by the Italian physician and poet Giralomo Fracastoro in his epic noted poem titled "Syphilis sive morbus gallicus". The first well-recorded European syphilis outbreak occured in 1494 during the siege of Naples by the French king Charles VIII (Hutto, 2001; Oriel, 1994; Bankl, 2002).

A worldwide spread of syphilis could then be observed. In scientific reports around the 19th century specific forms of neurosyphilis were grouped under the multicausal term "*Paralytic Dementia*". This term was defined as a syndrome, in which various forms of diseases such as syphilis, alcoholism, head injuries, hereditary diseases, and others were included. All of them presented demential and paralytical symptoms as common course (see graph 1). By the end of the 19th century approx. 45% of male patients hospitalized in psychiatric clinics in German speaking countries suffered from paralytic dementia. The number of patients suffering from neurosyphilis remains unclear. At the same time Emil Kraepelin reported that 34% of male patients suffered from a syphilis related paresis (Diefendorf, 1906).

In 1905, Schaudinn and Hoffmann discovered **Treponema pallidum** in tissue of patients with syphilis. One year later, the first effective test for Syphilis, the "Wassermann Test", was developed. In 1909, Nobel laureate Paul Ehrlich developed, together with his assistant Sahachiro Hata, Salvarsan, an arsenic compound, which is considered as the first effective treatment against syphilis before the penicillin era (Gensini et al, 2007). In 1913, Noguchi Hideyo demonstrated the presence of Treponema pallidum in the brain of progressive paralysis patients and was the first to establish a link between an infection with Treponema pallidum and the "Progressive paralysis" and "Tabes dorsalis" (Rulliere, 1992). The Austrian psychiatrist Julius Wagner Ritter von Jauregg tried inoculation of malaria parasites, which proved to be very successful in the case of dementia paralytica caused by neurosyphilis. It had been observed that patients who developed high fevers could be cured of syphilis as Treponema pallidum does not survive temperatures exceeding 41 ° C. In 1927, the discovery earned him the Nobel Prize in Physiology and Medicine (Nobel Lectures, 1965).

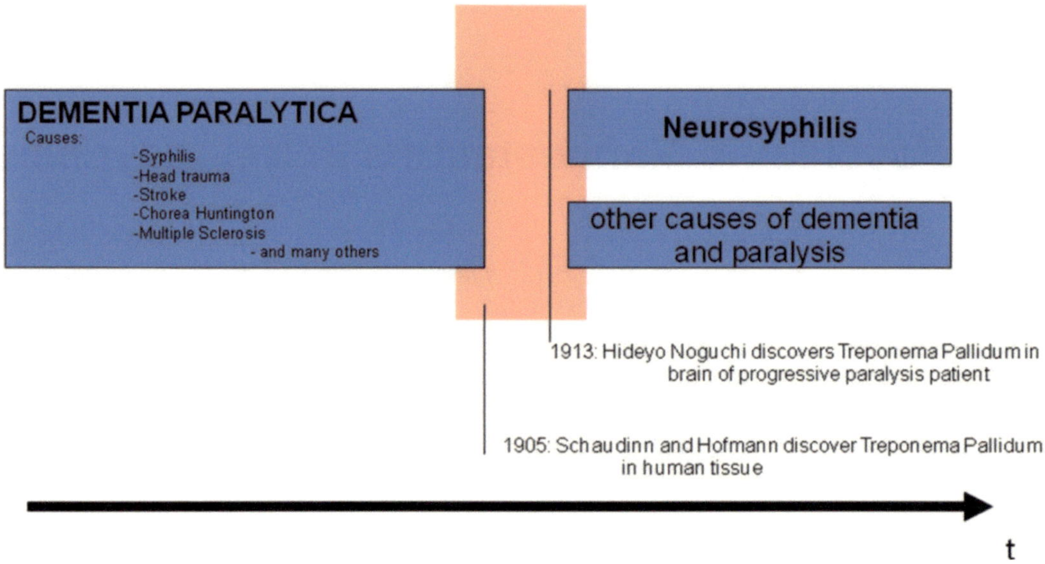

Graph 1. From the multicausal term „Dementia paralytica" to „Progressive paralysis" as a form of neurosyphilis

1.2 Epidemiological aspects

The dicscovery of penicillin and its widespread manufacture after World War II led to a decrease in syphilis infection rates. Until the 1990s syphilis has become a rare disease. Due to the low incidence a "syphilis eradication program" was planned by the Centers for Disease Control and Prevention (CDC) (Klausner et al, 2005). At present, it is obvious that the disease has not been eradicated. Estimations of the World Health Organization speak of 10-12 million new infections each year, primarily in developing countries of Africa and South America. Epidemiological data show a dramatic increase of infectious syphilis since the mid 1990s, mainly in the countries of the former Soviet Union, but also in Western European countries. A similar trend has been observed in the United States of America. According to recent epidemiological data rates of syphilis have been increasing in the United States and Europe, primarily among young adults and among men who have sex with men in urban areas or with individuals infected with HIV. It is important to mention, that the increase of syphilis prevalence is namely due to new infections (Lautenschlager, 2006; Geusau, 2004; Wöhrl, 2007).

1.3 Clinical aspects

Due to the variety of its clinical presentations syphilis is called the chameleon of diseases, potentially affecting every organ of the body. Therefore, it is easy to overlook the symptoms at any stage. All symptoms of secondary stage will resolve with or without treatment and the patient enters the asymptomatic latent period in which an infection can be detected only by laboratory diagnosis. Two thirds of these patients remain asymptomatic. If left untreated, years to decades after primary infection, up to 30% of the affected individuals may develop tertiary syphilis. Tertiary syphilis can manifest as benign gummas, as cardiovascular disease (e.g. aneurysm of the ascending aorta), or as neurosyphilis (Workowski & Berman, 2006; Wöhrl 2007).

However, the central nervous system may be involved already in the secondary stage. In this context the authors would like to refer to psychiatric manifestations of syphilitic arteriitis with secondary thrombosis (Berlit, 2006; Wöhrl, 2007).
Clinical manifestations of neurosyphilis can be divided into different subtypes (table 1).The asymptomatic form is characterized by the presence of a CNS infection as indicated by CSF abnormalities in the absence of psychiatric or other symptoms. Further, neurosyphilis is divided in a meningeal, a meningovascular, a parenchymatous, and a gummatous subform (Freedberg et al, 1999). This classification seems useful and is widely used (Flood et al, 1998, Friedrich et al, 2009).

I.	Asymptomatic		
II.	Meningeal		
	-	acute meningitis	
			-with hydrocephalus
			-with vertex involvement
			-with basiliar involvement
	-	spinal pachymeningitis	
III.	Meningovascular		
	-	cerebral	
	-	spinal	
			-meningomyelitis
			-acute transverse meningitis
IV.	Parenchymatous		
	-	general paresis	
	-	tabes dorsalis	
	-	optic atrophy	
V.	Gummatous		
	-	cerebral compression symptoms	
	-	spinal compression symptoms	

Table 1. Classification of neurosyphilis (Freedberg et al, 1999)

2. Psychiatric manifestations of neurosyphilis

Clinical manifestations as well as psychiatric symptoms of syphilis are diverse and have to be considered as non-specific. Table 2 gives an overview of psychiatric manifestations of neurosyphilis, classified according to the Tenth revision of the International Classification of Disease and Related Health Problems (= ICD-10) diagnoses.
Only few and inconsistent data about the prevalence of psychiatric manifestations of neurosyphilis can be found. In a retrospective analysis Timmermans et al (2004) report that approximately 51% of 161 patients diagnosed with neurosyphilis presented neuropsychiatric symptoms. A Danish study carried out over 17 years by Danielsen et al (2004) reports of 92 patients suffering of neurosyphilis: 36% of these patients initially presented with neurological symptoms, 17% with psychiatric manifestations.
Clinical manifestations of neurosyphilis are protean as stated above. A retrospective analysis of 117 patients by Flood et al (1998) shows a wide range of courses and symptoms

of neurosyphilis: 32% were asymptomatic, 33% presented personality changes, 28% of the patients had ataxia, 23% had a stroke, and 17% had ocular symptoms. 17 % of the patients reported bladder disturbance, whilst 10% had typical shooting pains due to tabes dorsalis. Headache, dizziness, or hearing loss was observed in 10% of the patients, 7% of the patients had cerebral seizures. Mitsonis et al (2008) examined medical records of 81 patients suffering from neurosyphilis. Between 1965-1984 approx. 27% of the individuals showed psychiatric manifestations, while between 1985-2005 almost 86% had psychiatric symptoms. The reason for this difference could not be explained by the authors.

Hoche (1912)	ICD-10: DD	Literatur
simple demential course	**F0: dementia**	Montejo et al 1995; Goeman et al 1996; Russouw et al 1997; Antonowicz 1998; Fox et al. 2000; Hutto et al 2000; Fujimoto et al 2001; Polsky et al 2001; Morikawa et al 2002; Xue et al 2004; Timmermans et al 2004; Blatz et al 2005; Lee et al 2005; Lessig et al 2006; Mahmoudi et al. 2006; Brinar et al 2006; Gabriel et al 2007; Van Eijsden et al 2008; Luo et al 2008; Lee et al 2009; Ates et al 2009; Mehrabian et al 2009; Yu et al 2010; Güler et al 2010
	F0:others	Zifko et al 1995; Russouw et al 1997; Boerner 1997; Flood et al 1998; Denays et al 1999; Mancuso et al 2000; Sobhan et al 2004; Ilankovic et al 2004; Lair et al 2004; Blatz et al 2005; Estevez 2006; Foatelli et al 2006; Sanchez et al 2007; Mannekote et al 2008; Tibrewal et al 2008
	F1	Cnossen et al 1995; Hutto et al 2000; Hutto 2001; Saik et al 2004; Blatz et al 2005; Yu et al 2009; Spiegel et al 2010
paranoid course	**F2**	Patkar et al 1997; Russouw et al 1997; Hutto et al 2000; Kohler et al. 2000; Kararizou et al 2006; Taycan et al 2006; Turan et al 2007; Friedrich et al. 2009
depressive course	**F3**	Zifko et al 1995; König et al 1996; Masmoudil et al 1996; Russouw et al 1997; Hutto et al 2000; Ide et al 2004; Blatz et al 2005; Mirsal et al 2007; Woo et al 2007; Cubała et al 2008
euphoric-expansive course	**F31: mania**	Bschor et al. 1995; Dawson & Baldwin 1996; Palicio et al 1996; Mimura et al 1997; Russouw et al 1997; Dunivin & Foust 1999; Kornischka 1999; Mendez 2000; Mahendran 2001; Spiegel et al 2010
	F4	Boyle et al 1995, Schreiber 1996; Aigner et al 1997; Hutto et al 2000
	F6	Zifko et al 1995; Tso et al 2008

(DD= differential diagnosis; F= ICD-10 Chapter V: Mental and behavioural disorders)

Table 2. Publications with psychiatric differential diagnosis of neurosyphilis according to ICD-10 compared to the classification of Hoche (1912);

In an earlier survey carried out by Hooshmand and colleagues (1972), data of 241 neurosyphilis patients were analysed for the period between 1965 and 1970. The majority of the patients presented with rather mild complaint forms of primarily peripheric neuropathic symptoms, while psychiatric manifestations seemed to be rare: 5% presented depression, 3% manic states and 2% presented personality changes.

Danielsen et al (2004) carried out another analysis of the various forms of neurosyphilis distinguishing between frequency and occurrence of psychiatric symptoms: 27% of patients were asymptomatic, while 10% were diagnosed with a meningovascular, 50 % with a parenchymatous, and 13% with a non-classifiable form of syphilis. Psychiatric manifestations could only be found in parenchymatous forms of neurosyphilis.

In his work from 1912, Hoche divides the course of psychopathological forms of progressive paralysis into an euphoric-expansive, a depressed, a paranoid, and a simple dementia onset form. This nomenclature is also found in today´s psychiatric textbooks as a valid classification. In this context Bonhoeffer´s axiom of non-specific noxa concerning organic psychosyndromes has to be mentioned: different kinds of primary or secondary affections of the brain can result in an organic brain syndrome, which does not seem to be differentiable in psychopathological terms. On the other hand, different types of organic brain syndromes can be found despite identical underlying somatic disease (Bonhoeffer, 1917). Table 2 shows a wider diagnostic spectrum with further progressions for psychiatric manifestations of neurosyphilis.

Analysing the psychopathological aspects with reference to the ICD-10 (see table 2) different kinds of manifestations of acute (e.g. amnestic passage syndrome), and chronic organic psychosyndromes (e.g. organic personality changes) can be observed. A great number of publications focus on demential syndromes (e.g. Yu et al, 2010; Ates et al, 2009). Goeman and colleagues (1996) for example report in their survey on the occurrence of dementia symptoms in a 15-year-old boy with congenital syphilis. Meteo-Ayuso´s (2000) recommendation for dementia symptoms accompanying syphilis is a symptomatic treatment with acetylcholinesterase inhibitors and / or memantines. Furthermore, various national Alzheimer societies recommend syphilis serologic testing as part of routine medical investigation of a demential syndrome (e.g. Schmidt et al, 2010).

A few case reports on substance dependence in association with neurosyphilis are available. Hutto (2001, 2000) reports of a patient initially treated for cocaine dependency, depression, and psychotic symptoms. Initial syphilis screening detected the eventual presence of neurosyphilis. Similar cases can be found for alcohol dependence (e.g. Cnossen et al, 1995; Blatz et al, 2005; Hutto, 2000). These cases show in particular the eventual co-incidence of a syphilis infection and psychiatric disorders.

Manifestations of syphilis with psychotic symptoms can vary from specific forms of hallucinations (e.g. Russouw et al, 1997) to various schizophrenia like symptoms (e.g. Kornischka, 1999; Friedrich et al, 2009). Some authors report of an improvement of psychotic symptoms after the initiation of causal penicillin therapy (e.g. Mannekote et al, 2008; Friedrich et al, 2009). However, it should be noted that the overall benefit of antibiotic therapy in advanced neuronal damage is limited. Only a few data is available on different antipsychotic treatment regimens for syphilitic psychotic state images: Turan er al (2007) carried out an evaluation of ziprasidone in comparison to olanzapine, Taykan et al (2006) the effect of quetiapine and risperidone. Furthermore, Rothenhäusler (2007) recommends the application of quetiapine and aripiprazole for the treatment of "syphilitic psychosis", in addition to antibiotic therapy.

Some publications report of mood disorders associated with neurosyphilis: depressive states (e.g. Frank et al, 1996) are described, as well as manic episodes (e.g. Mahendran et al, 2001). Rozwens and colleagues (2003) report that approx. 27% of patients with psychiatric manifestations of neurosyphilis presented depressive symptoms in association with psychomotoric retardation, melancholia, and suicidal thoughts.
The reader should be aware that apart from manifestations classified by the ICD-10-F further psychiatric-related manifestations of neurosyphilis may occur, such as epileptic seizures (eg, Gürses et al, 2007; Sinha et al, 2008), autism (eg, Blatz et al, 2005), paresis (eg, Chen et al, 2005), pain symptoms (Mao et al, 2009), parkinsonism (Spitz et al, 2008), and Huntington's chorea (Ozben et al, 2009).

3. Discussion and conclusion

In past decades, neurosyphilis has been perceived as a rare, almost forgotten and "historic disease". The rise of new infections with Treponema pallidum has confronted junior colleagues in the medical community with a variety of symptoms and manifestations that they have rarely seen in association with syphilis. Most of them have little knowledge of the complex appearance, the diagnosis, and the therapeutic options for this infectious disease (Aigner et al, 1997). The appropriate screening for syphilis in serum by Treponema antibody tests, such as the Treponema Pallidum Particle Agglutination Test (TPPA), is necessary to reveal a tertiary syphilis. These tests are, in particular for asymptomatic patients in the stage of late latency, the only reference to an infection with Treponema pallidum (Wöhrl, 2007). Depending on the activity of the illness indicated by high titers of nontreponemal tests, further evaluation for neurosyphilis by clinical and cerebrospinal fluid investigations is indicated. It is recommended that each patient with clinically evident psychiatric symptoms should have blood screening for syphilis - and in case of positive test results - a lumbar puncture.
The cost-benefit analysis of routine syphilis screening has been questioned in the recent past and current studies. In 2007, Cheng and colleagues (2007) emphasizes in terms of syphilis screening and intervention in 500.000 pregnant women the importance and efficacy of these tests. Recent epidemiological data show that syphilis is not only a problem of the so-called developing countries. There has been a recent increase of infection rates in industrialized countries of the Western world as well. Therefore, routine blood screening for syphilis in the psychiatric field remains a vital part of the investigation of psychiatric inpatients. Due to diversity of clinical manifestations of neurosyphilis (table 2) it is impossible to carry out a diagnosis only on the basis of clinical symptoms.
The Centers for Disease Control and Prevention (CDC) defines confirmed neurosyphilis as any syphilis stage and a reactive CSF-Venereal Disease Research Laboratory (VRDL). Further the CDC defines presumptive neurosyphilis as any syphilis stage, a nonreactive CSF-VDRL, an elevated CSF protein or white blood cell (WBC) count in the absence of other known causes of these abnormalities, and clinical symptoms or signs consistent with neurosyphilis without other known causes for these abnormalities (Centers for Disease Control and Prevention, 2010; Marra, 2009). Recommended therapy for neurosyphilis is the use of Aqueous crystalline penicillin G 18-24 million units per day, administered as 3-4 million units IV every 4 hours or continuous infusion, for 10-14 days. Furthermore, benzathine penicillin, 2.4 million units IM once per week up to 3 weeks are recommended after completion of the treatment regimen. If CSF pleocytosis was present initially, a CSF

examination should be repeated every 6 months until a normal cell count can be found. In the presence of a penicillin allergy, the use of ceftriaxone 2g daily (IV or IM) is suggested for 10-14 days as alternative treatment (Centers for Disease Control and Prevention, 2010).

Further, the authors would like to point out that there are no consensus and guidelines on how to deal with psychiatric manifestations in association with neurosyphilis (Sanchez et al, 2007). Therefore, an analysis of existing data and the initiation of prospective surveys are important for an effective and comprehensive treatment of affected patients in the future.

Psychiatrists play an essential role in the detection of syphilis and its late manifestations. Some authors (Hutto, 2001; Mirsal et al, 2007) state that psychiatric patients may have a higher risk to acquire syphilis during their lifetime. Impulse control dysfunctions, a high-risk sexual behavior, such as promiscuity or unprotected sex, or cognitive impairment and difficulties in seeking health care and assistance may be the cause for it.

Finally, there has to be a discussion on possibilities of co-morbidities in neurosyphilis and resulting difficulties in diagnosis. It often seems to be difficult to distinguish between pre-existing psychiatric disorders with secondary aggravation due to neurosyphilis and a secondary psychiatric disorder as a result of neurosyphilis. The situation gets even more complicated in the presence of a co-infection with HIV. Immunodeficiency may lead to a more rapid progression of syphilis to the stage of neurosyphilis, eventually with manifestations even a short time after infection (de Almeida et al, 2010; Marra, 2009).

4. Acknowledgement

No conflict of interest.

5. References

Aigner M, Ossege M, Bach M & Lenz G (1997). Indikationskriterien zum gezielten Luesscreening. *Nervenarzt;* 68: 752-753.

Antonowicz JL (1998). Missed diagnoses in consultation liaison psychiatry. *Psychiatr Clin North Am;* 21: 705-714.

Arbeitsgruppe für STD und dermatologische Mikrobiologie der österreichischen Gesellschaft für Dermatologie (2009). *Leitlinien zur Therapie der klassischen Geschlechtskrankheiten und Sexually Transmitted Infections;* www.oegdv.at

Ates MA, Algul A, Gecici O, Semiz UB, Yilmaz O & Gulsun M (2009). Olanzapine treatment in Jarish-Herxheimer reaction due to neurosyphilis with dementia: a case report. *J Psychopharmacol* 23: 999-1000.

Ayuso-Meteo JL (2000) Psychiatric aspects of infections. In: *New Oxford Textbook of Psychiatry,* Gelder MG, Lopez-Ibor JrJJ, Andreasen NC (eds) Vol 2, 1168-1173. Oxford.

Bankl H (2002) *Kolumbus brachte nicht nur die Tomaten.* Kremayr & Scheriau, Wien

Berlit P(2006) *Klinische Neurologie.* Springer Medizin Verlag, Heidelberg

Blatz R, Kühn HJ, Hermann W, Rytter M & Rodloff AC (2005) Neurosyphilis oder Neuroborreliose - retrospektive Auswertung von 22 Auswertungen. *Nervenarzt* 76: 724-732

Boerner RJ (1997) Organic psychosyndrome with progressive paralysis - a case report. *Nervenheilkunde* 16: 464-467.

Bonhoeffer K (1917) Die exogenen Reaktionstypen. *Arch Psychiatr Nervenkr* 58:58-70

Boyle A, Zafar R, Riley V & Lindesay J (1995) Neurosyphilis presenting with dissociative symptoms. *J Neurol Neurosurg Psychiatry* 59: 452-453.

Brinar VV & Habek M (2006) Dementia and white-matter demyelination in young patient with neurosyphilis. *Lancet* 368: 2258

Bschor T, Nurnbach-Ross B & Albrecht J (1995) Organic origin of manic psychosis. A case report of progressive paralysis. *Nervenarzt* 66: 54-56.

Centers for Disease Control and Prevention (2010) Sexually Transmitted diseases Treatment Guidelines, 2010. *MMWR* 59: RR12.

Chen CW, Chiang HC, Chen PL, Hsieh PF, Lee YC & Chang MH (2005) General paresis with reversible mesial temporal T2-weighted hyperintensity on magnetic resonance image: a case report. *Acta Neurol Taiwan* 14: 208-212.

Cheng JQ, Zhou H, Hong FC, Zhang D, Zhang YJ, Pan P et al (2007) Syphilis screening and intervention in 500 000 pregnant women in Shenzen, the People´s Republic of China. *Sex Transm Infect* 83: 347-350.

Cnossen WM, Niekus H, Nielson O, Vegt M & Blansjaar BA (1995) Cetriaxone treatment of penicillin resistant neurosyphilis in alcoholic patients. *J Neurol Neurosurg Psychiatry* 59: 194-195.

Cubala WJ & Czarnowska-Cubala M (2008) Neurosyphilis presenting with depressive symptomatology: is it unusual? *Acta Neuropsychiatr* 20: 110.

Danielsen AG, Weismann K, Jorgensen BB, Heidenheim M & Fugleholm AM (2004) Incidence, clinical presentation, and treatment of neurosyphilis in Denmark, 1980-1997. *Acta Derm Venereol* 84:459-462.

Dawson G & Baldwin B (1996). Neurosyphilis and secondary mania in elderly patients. *Ir J Psychol Med* 13: 24-25.

de Almeida SM, Bhatt A, Riggs PK, Durelle J, Lazaretto D, Marquie-Beck J, Mc Cutchan A, Letendre S & Ellis R (2010). Cerebrospinal fluid human immunodeficiency virus viral load in patients with neurosyphilis. *J Neurovirol* 16:6-12.

Denays R, Collier A, Rubinstein M & Atsama P (1999) A 51-year old woman with disorientation and amnesia. *Lancet* 354 : 1786.

Diefendorf AR (1906) Etiology of Dementia Paralytica. *BMJ* September; 744-748

Dunivin DL & Foust MJ (1999) A case study from the department of defense psychopharmacology demonstration project: mania and neurosyphilis. *Prof Psychol Res Pr* 30: 346-351.

Estevez RF (2006) Neurosyphilis presenting as rhabdomyolysis and acute renal failure with subsequent irreversible psychosis and dementia. *Psychosomatics* 47: 538-539

Flood JM, Weinstock HS, Guroy ME, Bayne L, Simon RP & Bolan G (1998) Neurosyphilis during the AIDS epidemic, San Francisco, 1985-1992. *J Infect Dis* 177: 931-940.

Foatelli FM, Gernay P, Lievens I & Ansseau M (2006) Syndrome malin der neuroleptiques et paralyse generale. *Rev Med Liege* 61: 807-811.

Fox PA, Hawkins DA & Dawson S (2000) Dementia following an acute presentation of meningovascular neurosyphilis in an HIV-1- positive patient. *Aids* 14: 2062-2063.

Frank U, Wolfersdorf M, Loble M & Hafele M (1996) Paranoide Depression bei progressiver Paralyse, Vitamin B-12 Mangel und subklinischer Hyperthyreose. *Nervenheilkunde* 15: 173-177.

Freedberg IM, Eisen A, Wolff K, Austen KF, Goldsmith LA, Katz S & Fitzpatrick T (1999). *Fitzpatrick´s Dermatology in General Medicine- Volume II.* Fifth Edition, Mc Graw-Hill. New York, San Francisco.

French P, Gomberg M, Janier M, Schmidt B, van Voorst Vader P & Young H (2009) IUSTI: 2008 European Guidelines on the Management of Syphilis. *Int J STD AIDS* 20 : 300-309.

Friedrich F, Geusau A, Greisenegger S, Ossege M & Aigner M (2009) Manifest psychosis in neurosyphilis. *Gen Hosp Psychiatry* 31:379-381.

Fujimoto H, Imaizumi T, Nishimura Y, Miura Y, Ayabe M, Shoji H & Abe T (2001) Neurosyphilis showing transient global amnesia-like attacks and magnetic resonance imaging abnormalities mainly in the limbic system. *Int Med* 40: 439-442.

Gabriel JP, Velon A, Ribeiro P, Santos MA & Silva MR (2007) Demential syndrome secondary to neurosyphilis. *Synapse* 7: 63-67.

Gensini GF, Conti AA & Lippi D (2007) The contributions of Paul Ehrlich to infectious disease. *J Infect* 54: 221-224.

Geusau A, Mayerhofer S, Schmidt B, Messeritsch E & Tschachler E (2004) The year 2002 re-emergence of syphilis in Austria. *Int J STD AIDS* 15:496-497.

Goeman J, Hoksbergen I, Pickut BA, Dom L, Crols R & De Deyn PP (1996) Dementia paralytica in a fifteen-year-old boy. *J Neurol Sci* 144 : 214-217.

Güler E & Leyhe T (2010) A late form of neurosyphilis manifesting with psychotic symptoms in old age and good response to ceftriaxone therapy. *International Psychogeriatrics*, article in press.

Gürses C, Kürtüncü M, Jirsch J, Yesilot N, Hanagasi H, Bebek N, Baykan B, Emre M, Gökyigit A & Andermann F (2007) Neurosyphilis presenting with status epilepticus. *Epileptic Disord* 9: 51-56.

Hoche A (1912) Dementia paralytica. In: *Handbuch der Psychiatrie* .Aschaffenburg G (Ed). Deuticke; Leipzig

Hooshmand H, Escobar MR & Kopf SW (1972) Neurosyphilis: a study of 241 patients. *JAMA* 219:726-729.

Hutto B & Adimora A (2000) Syphilis in Psychiatric Inpatients: prevalence, treatment and implications. *Gen Hosp Psychiatry* 22:291-293.

Hutto B (2001) Syphilis in clinical psychiatry. *Psychosomatics* 42: 453-460

Ide M, Mizukami K, Fujita T, Ashizawa Y & Asada T (2004) A case of neurosyphilis showing a marked improvement of clinical symptoms and cerebral blood flow on single photon emission computed tomography with quantitative penicillin treatment. *Prog Neuropsychopharmacol Biol Psychiatry* 28: 417-420.

Ilankovic N, Ivkovic M, Sokic D, Ilankovic A, Milovanovic S, Filipovic B, Tiosavljevic D, Ilankovic V & Bojic V (2004) Dementia paralytica (neurosyphilis): a clinical case study. *World J Biol Psychiatry* 4: 135-138.

Kararizou E, Mitsonis C, Dimopoulos N, Gkiatas K, Markou I & Kalfakis N (2006) Psychosis or simply a new manifestation of neurosyphilis? *J Int Med Res* 34: 335-337.

Klausner JD, Kent CK, Wong W, McCright J & Katz MH (2005) The public health response to epidemic syphilis, San Francisco, 1999-2004. *Sex Transm Dis* 32:S11-S18.

Kohler CG, Pickholtz J & Ballas C (2000) Neurosyphilis presenting as schizophrenialike psychosis. *Neuropsychiatry Neuropsychol Behav Neurol* 13: 297-302.

König F, Frank U, Wolfersdorf M, Löble M & Häfele M (1996) Paranoide Depression bei progressive Paralyse, Vitmain B-12Mangel und subklinishcer Hyperthyreose. *Nervenheilkunde* 15: 173-177.

Kornischka J (1999) Maniforme Psychose bei Neurolues. *Psych Prax* 26: 256.

Lair L & Naidech AM (2004) Modern neuropsychiatric presentation of neurosyphilis. *Neurol* 63: 1331-1333

Lautenschlager S (2006) Syphilisdiagnostik: Klinische und labormedizinische Problematik. *JDDG* 12: 1058-1073.

Lee CH, Lin WC, Lu CH & Liu JW (2009) Initially unrecognized dementia in a young man with neurosyphilis. *Neurologist* 15: 95-97

Lee JW, Wilck M & Venna N (2005) Dementia due to neurosyphilis with persistently negative CSF VDRL. *Neurol* 65 : 1838

Lessig S & Tecoma E (2006) Perils of the prozone reaction: neurosyphilis presenting as an RPR-negative subacute dementia. *Neurol* 66: 777

Luo W, Ouvang Z, Xu H, Chen J, Ding M & Zhang B (2008) The clinical analysis of general paresis with 5 cases. *Neuropsychiatry Clin Neurosci* 20: 490-493

Mahendran R (2001) Clozapine in the treatment of hypomania with neurosyphilis. *J Clin Psychiatry* 62 : 477-478

Mahmoudi R, Maheut-Bosser A, Hanesse B & Paille F (2006) La Neurosyphilis: une cause rare de démence. *Rev Med Interne* 27: 976-978

Mancuso A, Sbrana R, Ghersi L, Bernareggi N & Gorini M (2000) Neurosyphilis: an atypical case. *Neurol Sci* 21: S165-S166

Mannekote ST & Singh VK (2008) A case of neurosyphilis presenting with treatment-resistant psychotic symptoms and progressive cognitive dysfunction. *Ger J Psychiatr* 11: 153-155

Mao S, Liu Z (2009) Neurosyphilis manifesting as lightning pain. *Eur J Dermatol* 19: 504-506

Marra CM (2009) Update on Neurosyphilis. *Curr Infect Dis Rep* 11:127-134

Masmoudil K, Joly H, Rosa A & Mizon JP (1996) Does general paresis always exist in non-AIDS patient ? *Rev Med Int* 17: 576-578

Mehrabian S, Raycheva MR, Petrova EP, Tsankov NK & Traykov LD (2009) Neurosyphilis presenting with dementia, chronic chorioretinitis and adverse reactions to treatment : a case report. *Cases J* 2: 8334

Mendez MF (2000) Mania in neurologic disorders. *Curr Psychiatry Rep* 2: 440-445.

Mimura M, Kato M, Ishii K, Yoshino F, Saito F & Kashima H (1997) A neuropsychological and neuroimaging study of a patient before and after treatment of paretic neurosyphilis. *Neurocase* 3: 275-283

Mirsal H, Kalyoncu A, Pektas Ö & Beyazyürek M (2007) Neurosyphilis presenting as psychiatric symptoms: an unusual case report. *Acta Neuropsychiatr* 19: 251-253

Mitsonis CH, Kararizou E, Dimopoulos N, Triantafyllou N, Kapaki E, Mitropoulos P, Sfagos K & Vassilopoulos D (2008) Incidence and clinical presentation of Neurosyphilis: a retrospective study of 81 cases. *Int J Neurosci* 118: 1251-1257

Montejo M, Ruiz-Irastorza G, Aguirrebengoa, Onate K & Aurrekoetxea J (1995) Neurosyphilis as a cause of dementia: does it still exist ? *J Infect* 30: 186-187

Morikawa M, Kosaja J, Imai T, Ohsawa H, Iida J & Kishimoto T (2002) A case of general paresis showing marked treatment-associated improvement of cerebellar blood flow by quantitative imaging analysis. *Ann Nucl Med* 16: 71-74

Nobel Lectures (1965), Physiology or Medicine 1922-1941: Wagner-Jauregg J. *The Treatment of Dementia Paralytica by Malaria Inoculation*. Elsevier Publishing Company; Amsterdam

Oriel JD (1994) *The scars of Venus: A History of Venereology*. Springer Verlag: London.

Ozben S, Erol C, Ozer F & Tiras R (2009) Chorea as the presenting feature of neurosyphilis. *Neurol India* 57 : 347-349

Palicio L & Basauri VA (1996) Neurosyphilis with psychiatric manifestations - a forgotten condition? *Ir J Psychol Med* 13: 26-27

Patkar AA, Peng AT & Alexander RC (1997) Neurosyphilis occuring in a patient with schizohrenia: a cautionary tale. *J Nerv Ment Dis* 185 : 119-120.

Polsky I & Samuels SC (2001) Neurosyphilis: Screening does sometimes reveal an infectious cause of dementia. *Geriatrics* 56: 61-62

Rothenhäusler HB (2007) Neurosyphilis - Diagnose und Therapie vor psychiatrischem Hintergrund. *Fortschr Neurol Psychiatr* 75:737-747

Rozwens A, Radziwillowicz P, Jakuszkowiak K & Cubala WJ (2003) Neurosyphilis with its psychopathological implications. *Psychiatr Pol* 37:477-494

Rulliere R (1992) Die japanische Medizin. In: R. Toellner: *Illustrierte Geschichte der Medizin*. Andreas Verlag; Salzburg.

Russouw HG, Roberts MC, Emsley RA & Truter R (1997) Psychiatric manifestations and magnetic resonance imaging in HIV-negative neurosyphilis. *Biol Psychiatry* 41: 467-473

Saik S, Kraus JE, McDonald A, Mann SG & Sheitman BB (2004) Neurosyphilis in newly admitted psychiatric patients: three case reports. *J Clin Psychiatry* 65: 919-921

Sanchez FM & Zisselman MH (2007) Treatment of psychiatric symptoms associated with neurosyphilis. *Psychosomatics* 48: 440-445

Schmidt R, Marksteiner J, Dal Bianco P, Ransmayr G, Bancher C, Benke T, Wancata J, Fischer P, Leblhuber CF et al (2010) Konsensusstatement „Demenz 2010" der Österreichischen Alzheimer Gesellschaft. *Neuropsychiatr* 24: 67-87

Schreiber W (1996) Ein Fall von "Syphilitischer Neurasthenie". Zur neuen Brisanz eines fast vergessenen Chamäleons. *Psych Prax* 23 : 98-99

Sinha S, Harish T, Taly AB, Murthy P, Nagarathna S & Chandramuki A (2008) Symptomatic seizures in neurosyphilis: an experience from a university hospital in south India. *Seizure* 17: 711-716

Sobhan T, Rowe HM, William GR & Munoz C (2004) Three cases of psychiatric manifestations of neurosyphilis. *Psychiatr Serv* 55 : 830-832

Spiegel DR, Weller AL, Pennell K & Turner K (2010) The successfull treatment of mania due to acquired immunodeficiency syndrome using ziprasidone. *Journal of Neuropsychiatry and Clinical Neurosciences* 22 : 111-114

Spitz M, Maia FM, Gomes HR, Scaff M & Barbosa ER (2008) Parkinsonism secondary to neurosyphilis. *Mov Disord* 23: 1948-1949

Taycan O, Ugur M & Ozmen M (2006) Quetiapine vs. risperidone in treating psychosis in neurosyphilis: a case report. *Gen Hosp Psychiatry* 28: 359-361

Tibrewal P, Kumar I, Zutshi A & Math SB (2008) Valproate for treatment of agitation in neurosyphilis: a case report. *Prim Care Companion J Clin Psychiatry* 10: 163

Timmermans M & Carr J (2004) Neurosyphilis in the modern era. *J Neurol Neurosurg Psychiatry* 75: 1727-1730

Tso MK, Koo K & Tso GY (2008) Neurosyphilis in a non-HIV patient: more than a psychiatric concern. *Mcgill J Med* 11: 160

Turan S, Emul M, Duran A, Mert A & Ugur M (2007) Effectiveness of olanzapine in neurosyphilis related organic psychosis. A case report. *J Psychopharmacol* 21: 556-558

Van Eijsden P, Veldink JH, Linn FH, Scheltens P & Biessels GJ (2008) Progressive dementia and mesiotemporal atrophy on brain MRI: Neurosyphilis mimicking pre-senile Alzheimer´s disease. *Eur J Neurol* 15: e14-e15

Wöhrl S & Geusau A (2007) Clinical update: syphilis in adults. *Lancet* 369: 1912-1914

Woo B, Jeevarakshagan S, Sevilla C & Obrocea G (2007) Psychiatric and neuro-ophtalmological manifstations of syphilis. *Psychosomatics* 48 : 451

Workowski KA & Berman SM (2006) Sexually transmitted diseases treatment guidelines. *MMWR Recomm Rep* 55: 1-94

Xue XY & Meng SY (2004) Epidemiological analysis of reversible dementia in an outpatient department of neurology. *Chin J Clin Rehab* 8: 5388-5390

Yu Y, Wei M, Huang Y, Jiang W, Liu X, Xia F, Li D & Zhao G (2010) Clinical presentation and imaging of general paresis due to neurosyphilis in patients negative for human immunodeficiency virus. *J Clin Neurosci* 17: 308-310

Zifko U, Schmidt B, Grisold B & Stanek G (1995) Neurosyphilis - a case report and review of the literature concerning the differential diagnosis to Lyme borreliosis. *Wien Med Wochenschr* 145 : 191-194

5

Spatial and Temporal Patterns of Primary Syphilis and Secondary Syphilis in Shenzhen, China

Tiejian Feng, Yufeng Hu, Xiaobing Wu and Fuchang Hong
Shenzhen Center for Chronic Disease Control
China

1. Introduction

Syphilis remains a global problem with an estimated population of 12 million infected each year, despite the existence of effective prevention measures, such as condoms, and effective and relatively inexpensive treatment options (World Health Organization, Department of Reproductive Health and Research, 2007). China is currently witnessing a major resurgence of syphilis from the elimination of the disease in the 1960s to 8.7 cases per 100,000 people in 2005 (Chen et al., 2007). The total incidence of syphilis in 2009 was 24.66 cases per 100,000 people, with incidence of primary and secondary syphilis accounting for 11.74 cases per 100 000 people (National Center for STD control, CDC, China, 2009).

Shenzhen, a city located in southern coastal China and adjacent to Hong Kong, is also with great disease burden of syphilis. Preliminary estimation showed that there were more than 80,000 syphilis cases in Shenzhen (Hong et al., 2009a). A total of 22861 syphilis cases were reported from 2004 to 2008 in Shenzhen, ranking the first among 21 cities in Guangdong province. The total incidence was 73.07 cases per 100,000 people in 2008, which was 3.47 times higher than that in China and 2.19 times higher than that in Guangdong Province. Syphilis has become a very serious problem of public health in Shenzhen.

Population-based studies showed that lots of human factors were associated with genotype clustering in syphilis, including marital status, education level, age structure, human immunodeficiency virus (HIV) infection, homelessness, drug abuse and the local pornography (Newell et al., 1993). The local health bureau had paid much attention to syphilis prevention and control, and it set up a long-term program titled *Syphilis Prevention of Mother-to-Child Transmission* which had yielded great cost effect and largely reduced the incidence of congenital syphilis (Cheng et al., 2007; Hong et al., 2010; Cai et al., 2007). However, the total incidence of syphilis as well as the prevalence of syphilis among some high risk population (e.g., men who have sex with men) had been rising (Feng et al., 2008; Hong et al., 2009b). Actually, tens of health centers in Shenzhen had offered free voluntary counseling and testing for syphilis as well as HIV, and health education and promotion programs had been conducting, while the effects seemed limited. Then questions arose, had the prevention and intervention been put into the right place? Were there any clusters of syphilis? It was believed that if we could find out these clusters and encourage more intervention in these regions, it would largely reduce the incidence of syphilis. Explore the

genotype clusters of syphilis and describe its spatial and temporal patterns would be useful and it would provide essential information for designing syphilis intervention programs.
It used to be very difficult to decide which districts and what time the clusters would occur. If we simply compared the incidence of each district and/or each time period, it would be likely to cause selection bias as the spatial and temporal boundaries of the clusters had been set at the very beginning. Moreover, any geographical region always contained high-rate areas that occurred by chance alone. Using this method to find out the significant clusters needed to consider a lot of random variables, otherwise the statistics results would be far from truth (Kulldorff et al., 1998).
To solve the problem, Kulldorf and Nagarwalla advocated the generalized mathematical model to describe spatial distribution (Wallenstein, 1980). The model applied the likelihood ratio test, adjusted the underlying spatial in homogeneity of a background population and created the scan window with varied sizes to do the data statistics. Afterwards, Kulldor raised spatial scan statistics, space-time permutation scan statistics and prospective space-time permutation scan statistics which were based on Monte Carlo hypothesis test. Kulldorf and his colleagues also created SaTScan (available online for free at: http://www.satscan.org/) for the above statistics. This method was widely used to detect and evaluate disease clusters for a variety of diseases, including cancer (Jackson et al., 2009; Meliker et al., 2009), shigella infection (Stelling et al., 2009), malaria (Haqua et al., 2009; Coleman et al., 2009), low birth weight and infant mortality (Grady & Enander, 2009), amyotrophic lateral sclerosis (Scott et al., 2009) and diabetes (Green et al., 2003). Prospective space-time clustering statistics could also be used for early warning. This method might detect the outbreak at any place and any size as early as possible, which would facilitate public health officers to conduct related investigations and control program with the goal of preventing disease transmission (Kulldorff et al., 2005). Moreover, the prospective space-time permutation scan statistics could detect the abnormity in the process of disease transmission. Thus, it was widely used in acute infectious diseases and biological terror warning study (Kulldorff et al., 2005).
As the patients in primary and secondary syphilis stage would have higher transmission ratio, timely treatment and intervention among these cases would be more effective in syphilis prevention. Thus, this study aimed to identify the clusters of primary and secondary syphilis in Shenzhen in recent years via spatial and space-time statistics and detect the early warning signals of syphilis outbreak by prospective space–time permutation scan statistics.

2. Methods

2.1 Data sources

Data of syphilis cases was downloaded from the *China Information System for Disease Control and Prevention*. Patients' gender, date of birth, date of diagnosis, current address and other information (e.g., education level, marital status, occupation) were recorded in the database. Geographic Information System (GIS) data was from Shenzhen 1:10,000 digital maps. Data of population size was from the Shenzhen Municipal Bureau of Statistics.

2.2 Data coding

Shenzhen was divided into 55 neighbourhoods (the smallest administrative unit in Shenzhen). In this study, current address was recoded into 55 street communities which were matched with Shenzhen's GIS data. Date of diagnosis for each case was recoded by year.

2.3 Software and spatio-temporal clustering analysis

The spatio-temporal clustering analysis was carried out via SaTScan software. The purely spatial scan statistics imposes a circle window on the map. The window is in turn centered on each of several possible grid points positioned throughout the study region. For each grid point, the radius of the window varies continuously in size from zero to some upper limit defined by the user. In this way, the method creates lots of distinct geographical circles with different sets of neighboring data locations within them. Each circle is a possible candidate cluster (Kulldorff Martin. SaTScanTM User Guide for version 9.0. 2010.).

The space-time scan statistics is defined by a cylindrical window with a circular geographic base and with height corresponding to time. The base is defined exactly as for the purely spatial scan statistics, while the height reflects the time period of potential clusters. The cylindrical window is then moved in space and time. It creates a number of overlapping cylinders of different size and shape, jointly covering the entire study region, where each cylinder reflects a possible cluster (Kulldorff Martin. SaTScanTM User Guide for version 9.0. 2010.).

For each scanning window, the analysis process will firstly get the expected number of cases based on the observed number of cases, then calculate the log likelihood ratio (LLR) by observed number and expected number of cases inside or outside the window. LLR is used to evaluate the cluster status. The likelihood function is maximized over all window locations and sizes, and the one with maximum likelihood constitutes the most likely cluster. The likelihood ratio for this window constitutes the maximum likelihood ratio test statistics. Its distribution under the null-hypothesis is obtained by repeating the same analytic exercise on a large number of random replications of the data set generated under the null hypothesis. The *P*-value is obtained through Monte Carlo hypothesis testing, by comparing the rank of the maximum likelihood from the real data set with the maximum likelihoods from the random data sets. If this rank is R, then P=R/(1+simulation). In this study, the number of simulations is defined as 999, thus, the calculation of *P* value is accurate to three decimal.

For purely spatial and space-time analyses, it also identifies secondary clusters besides the most likely cluster, and orders them according to their likelihood ratio test statistic. There will always be a secondary cluster that is almost identical with the most likely cluster and that have almost high likelihood value, since expanding or reducing the cluster size only marginally with not change the likelihood very much. Most clusters of this type provide little additional information, but their existence indicates the possibility of pinpointing the general location of a cluster. There are some secondary clusters that do not overlap with the most likely cluster which are of great interest. In this study, we used the default settings, it means there was no geographical overlap between secondary clusters and the most likely clusters.

3. Results

A total of 9126 primary and secondary syphilis cases were reported from 2005 to 2008, with 5173 males and 3953 females (Table 1).

Year	Number of neighbourhood	Number of primary and secondary syphilis cases		
		Total	Male	Female
2005	55	2117	1162	955
2006	55	2364	1291	1073
2007	55	2211	1238	973
2008	55	2434	1482	952
Total		9126	5173	3953

Table 1. Primary and secondary syphilis cases reported from 2005 to 2008 in Shenzhen

3.1 Results of retrospective spatial scan statistics

In 2005, there were 12 statistically significant clusters ($P \le 0.05$), and two minor significant clusters ($P > 0.05$), while the numbers were eight and seven in 2006, ten and five in 2007, and nine and four in 2008 (Table 2-5). The distribution of clusters changed with years (See Figure 1). The neighbourhood with cluster number '1' was the most likely cluster. Other neighbourhoods which were not shown in Table 2-5 or with white color in Figure 1 were not clusters.

Cluster number	Neighbourhood	Actual incidence	Theory incidence	RR	*P* values
1	Longhua	101	31.28	3.34	≤0.001
2	Cuizhu	53	9.70	5.58	≤0.001
3	Huafu	72	19.32	3.82	≤0.001
4	Nanshan	153	69.08	2.31	≤0.001
4	Nantou	153	69.08	2.31	≤0.001
5	Lianhua	79	36.06	2.24	≤0.001
6	Guiyuan	69	34.96	2.01	≤0.001
6	Dongmen	69	34.96	2.01	≤0.001
7	Xin'an	96	58.54	1.67	≤0.001
8	Xixiang	109	70.25	1.58	≤0.001
9	Gongming	88	56.04	1.60	0.003
10	Futian	115	83.63	1.40	0.021
11	Songgang	71	55.20	1.30	0.769
12	Nanhu	22	13.72	1.61	0.771

Table 2. The significant and minor significant clusters in Shenzhen in 2005 by retrospective spatial scan statistics.

Cluster number	Neighbourhood	Actual incidence	Theory incidence	RR	*P* values
1	Cuizhu	100	10.83	9.59	≤0.001
2	Longhua	141	34.93	4.23	≤0.001
3	Lianhua	137	40.27	3.55	≤0.001
4	Huafu	94	21.57	4.50	≤0.001
5	Huangbei	104	44.42	2.40	≤0.001
5	Nanhu	104	44.42	2.40	≤0.001
6	Xin'an	117	65.38	1.83	≤0.001
7	Shekou	45	17.65	2.58	≤0.001
8	Nanshan	105	77.14	1.38	0.079
8	Nantou	105	77.14	1.38	0.079
9	Longgang	91	67.24	1.37	0.177
10	Songgang	81	61.64	1.33	0.484
11	Futian	116	93.39	1.25	0.553
12	Guiyuan	54	39.04	1.39	0.569
12	Dongmen	54	39.04	1.39	0.569

Table 3. The significant and minor significant clusters in Shenzhen in 2006 by retrospective spatial scan statistics.

Cluster number	Neighbourhood	Actual incidence	Theory incidence	RR	*P* values
1	Huafu	82	20.18	4.18	≤0.001
2	Nanhu	68	14.33	4.87	≤0.001
3	Cuizhu	54	10.13	5.44	≤0.001
4	Futian	186	87.35	2.23	≤0.001
5	Longhua	70	32.67	2.18	≤0.001
6	Dongmen	39	17.47	2.25	≤0.001
7	Shekou	37	16.51	2.26	≤0.001
8	Xixiang	110	73.37	1.53	0.002
9	Nanshan	107	72.15	1.51	0.005
9	Nantou	107	72.15	1.51	0.005
10	Mingzhi	43	30.57	1.41	0.709
11	Donghu	34	24.81	1.38	0.954
12	Xin'an	75	61.14	1.23	0.960
13	Dapeng	14	8.73	1.61	0.985
14	Lianhua	47	37.66	1.25	0.998

Table 4. The significant and minor significant clusters in Shenzhen in 2007 by retrospective spatial scan statistics.

Cluster number	Neighbourhood	Actual incidence	Theory incidence	RR	*P* values
1	Huafu	102	22.21	4.75	≤0.001
2	Cuizhu	73	11.15	6.72	≤0.001
3	Dongmen	213	96.16	2.33	≤0.001
4	Huangbei	127	45.73	2.87	≤0.001
4	Nanhu	127	45.73	2.87	≤0.001
5	Nantou	86	33.27	2.64	≤0.001
6	Longhua	82	35.96	2.32	≤0.001
7	Shekou	49	18.17	2.73	≤0.001
8	Donghu	46	19.23	2.42	≤0.001
9	Gongming	90	64.43	1.41	0.073
10	Xin'an	84	67.31	1.26	0.832
11	Lianhua	54	41.46	1.31	0.903
12	Songgang	75	63.46	1.19	0.994

Table 5. The significant and minor significant clusters in Shenzhen in 2008 by retrospective spatial scan statistics.

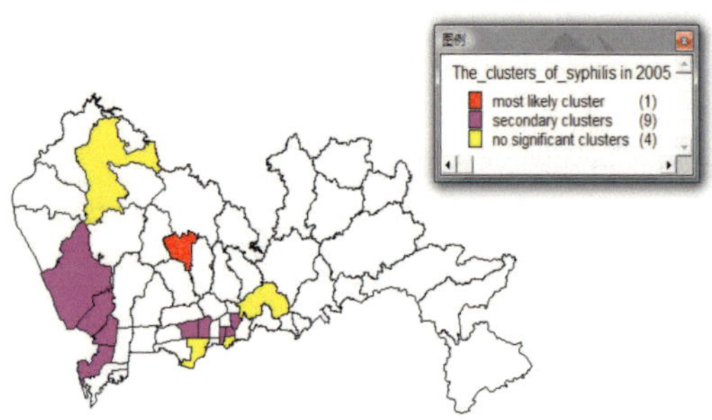

(a) Clusters in 2005

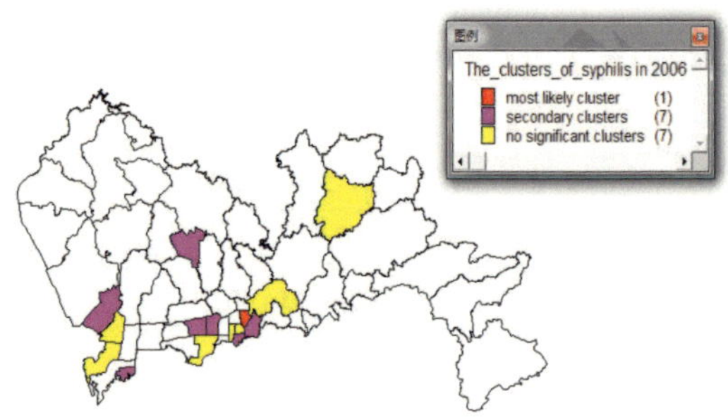

(b) Clusters in 2006

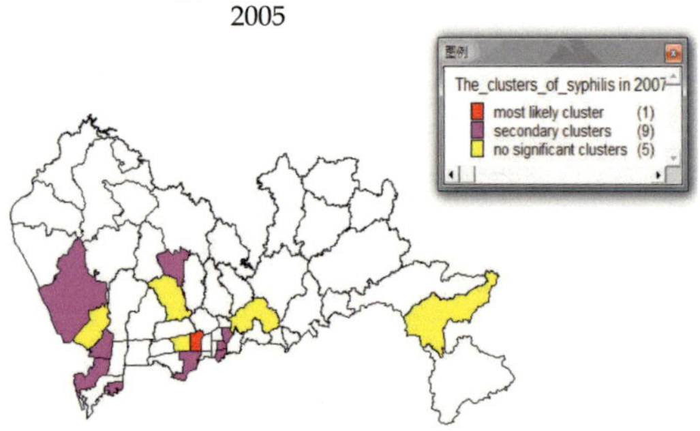

(c) Clusters in 2007

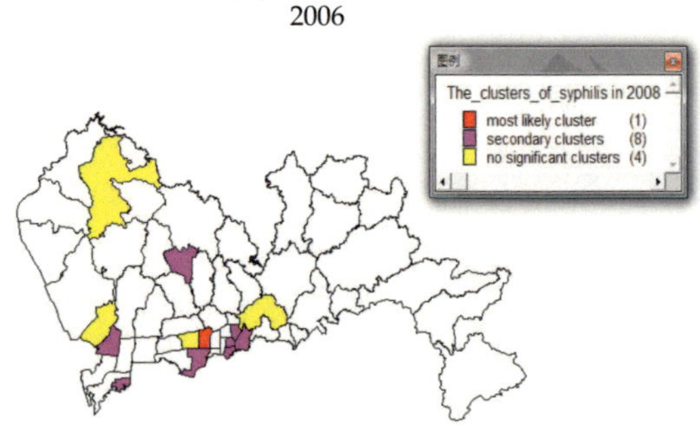

(d) Clusters in 2008

Fig. 1. Clusters of primary and secondary syphilis in Shenzhen by spatial scan statistics from 2005 to 2008

Throughout the study period (from 2005 to 2008), there were totally 15 clusters, among which Longhua, Cuizhu and Fuhua neighbourhoods were significant clusters in all the four study years. Five districts were significant clusters in three of the four study years (Figure 2).

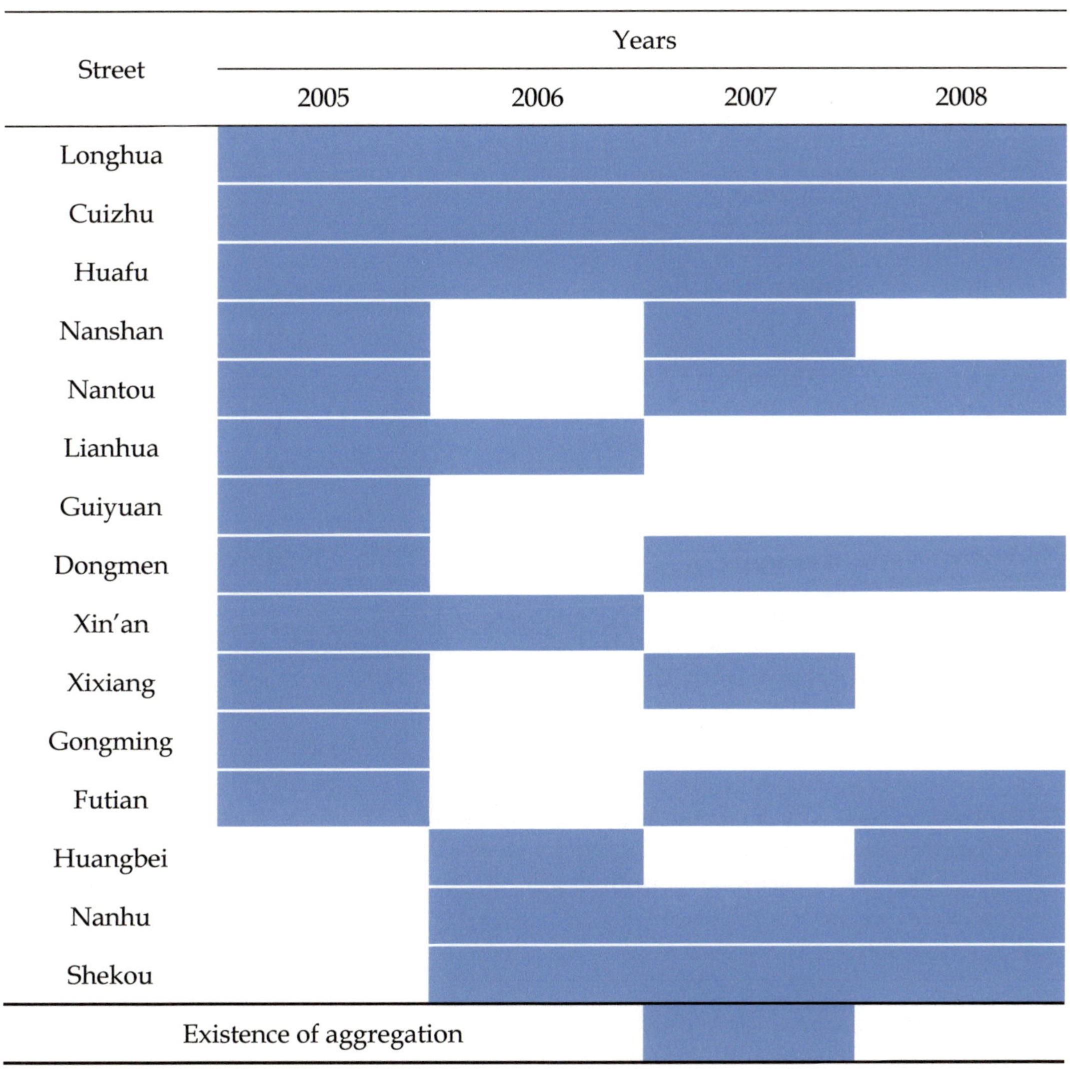

*Blue color=cluster, blank color=no cluster

Fig. 2. Temporal change of significant syphilis clusters, Shenzhen, 2005-2008, by purely spatial cluster analysis*

In this study, many minor statistically significant clusters became significant clusters in the following year or subsequent years, while some significant clusters became nonsignificant clusters conversely. The change of minor significant clusters also reflected the spatial and temporal trends (See Table 6).

Districts	Neighbourhood	2005	2006	2007	2008
1	Songgang	0	0	-1	0
2	Nanhu	0	1	1	1
3	Nanshan	1	0	1	-1
4	Nantou	1	0	1	1
5	Longgang	-1	0	-1	-1
6	Futian	1	0	1	1
7	Guiyuan	1	0	-1	-1
8	Dongmen	1	0	1	1
9	Mingzhi	-1	-1	0	-1
10	Donghu	-1	-1	0	-1
11	Xin'an	1	1	0	0
12	Dapeng	-1	-1	0	-1
13	Lianhua	1	-1	0	0
14	Gongming	1	-1	-1	0
15	Guanlan	-1	-1	-1	-1
16	Shekou	-1	1	1	1

Note: 1=the existence of statistically significant clusters in a certain year, 0=the existence of minor significant clusters in a certain year, -1=no cluster in a certain year.

Table 6. Changes of nonsignificant syphilis clusters from 2005 to 2008

3.2 Results of space-time permutation scan statistics

This study set the maximum spatial cluster size at 10 kilometers and the longest duration was two years. By space-time permutation scan statistics, ten significant clusters were detected in Shenzhen from 2005 to 2008, which was similar with the results of spatial scan statistics. See table 7 and Figure 3.

3.3 Early warning signal for syphilis outbreak

We explored the adaptability of prospective space-time scan statistics via analyzing the syphilis cases from Nov to Dec, 2005. The time span was set as 1 day, the maximum time window was 7 days (due to the early warning, time scale cannot be too long) and the greatest scanning radius was 10 kilometers. As patients would choose varied day of a week to visit the medical institutions (for example, many people would prefer to visit on Saturday and Sunday as they needed to work from Monday to Friday), this study adjusted the space by day-of-week interaction. By prospective space-time scan statistics, five early warning signals were found. The most likely clusters were located in Shekou and Zhaoshang with the recurrence interval of one year and 135 days (Table 8).

Cluster number	Neighbourhood	Time frame	Actual incidence	Theory incidence	*P* Values
1	Mingzhi	2007-2008	101	51.39	≤0.001
1	Bantian	2007-2008	101	51.39	≤0.001
2	Lianhua	2006	137	82.15	≤0.001
3	Dalang	2007—2008	41	20.86	≤0.001
4	Longhua	2006	141	102.11	0.004
5	Zhaoshang	2005	39	22.51	0.027
6	Hanggang	2007	113	82.89	0.028
7	Cuizhu	2006	100	72.56	0.039
8	Huangbei	2007—2008	249	205.03	0.048
8	Nanhu	2007—2008	249	205.03	0.048

Table 7. Location of statistically significant ($P \leq 0.05$) syphilis clusters, in Shenzhen, 2005-2008, by space-time permutation statistics.

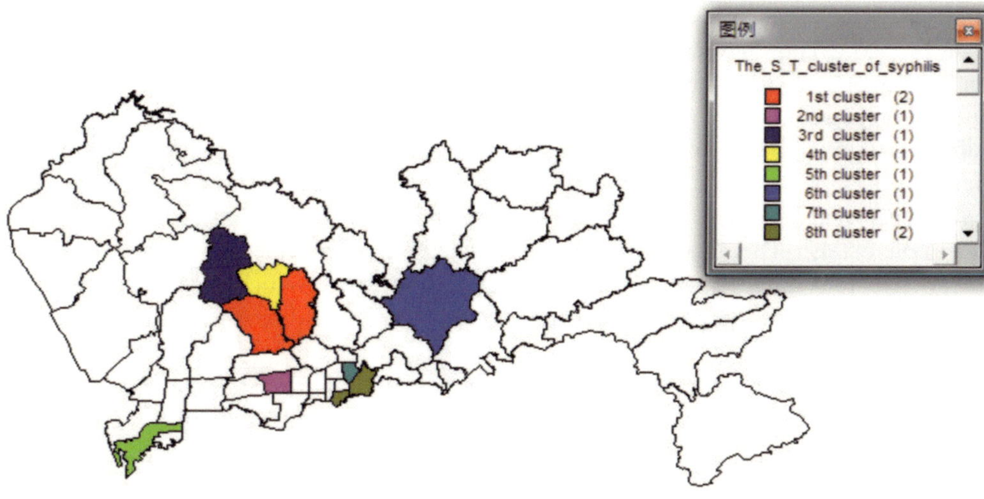

Fig. 3. Statistically significant clusters of syphilis in Shenzhen by space-time permutation scan statistics from 2005 to 2008.

Cluster number	Neighbourhood	Period of warning cluster	Actual incidence	Theory incidence	*P* Values	Recurrence interval
1	Shekou	2005/12/26 - 2005/12/31	9	2.07	0.002	1 year 135 days
1	Zhaoshang	2005/12/26 - 2005/12/31	9	2.07	0.002	1 year 135 days
2	Guanlan	2005/12/26 - 2005/12/31	8	2.09	0.021	48 days
3	Fuyong	2005/12/30 - 2005/12/31	8	2.11	0.022	45 days
3	Shajing	2005/12/30 - 2005/12/31	8	2.11	0.022	45 days

*: only shows the cluster of P≤0.05

Table 8. Early warning signals for primary and secondary syphilis in Shenzhen by prospective space-time permutation scan statistics*

4. Discussion

Identification of primary and secondary syphilis clusters can contribute to syphilis control strategies selection. Two different methods are applied in this study to explore the spatial and temporal patterns of primary and secondary syphilis in Shenzhen from 2005 to 2008. By purely spatial analysis, minor significant changes of the clusters' locations are found from 2005 to 2008. The clusters mainly concentrate in the neighbourhoods of Longhua, Xixiang, Xin'an, Nanshan, Nantou, Shekou, Futian, Fuhua, Cuizhu, Dongmen and Huangbei. Many of these neighbourhoods are adjacent to each other and most of them own large number of migrant workers as well as entertainment venues. A lot of surveys have proved that migrant workers are more likely to have unprotected sex behavior as their low risk perception, lack of money and psychological problem, resulting in more risk of syphilis infection. Moreover, the entertainment venues in these neighbourhoods meet the desire of migrant workers and encourage their sex behavior. Thus, the clusters of syphilis detected in this study may be associated with the clusters of high risk groups. More attention should be paid to the cluster areas. To accelerate progress towards epidemiological impact target sites, we should move up local government and public health agenda with increased resource allocation and enhance the intervention and prevention work.

The purely spatial analysis also shows the small-scale changes of syphilis clusters during the four study years. This may indicate the changes of syphilis incidence in the districts and reflect the changes of risk factors. But how the specific risk factors changed has not been discussed here, and it will be the topic of our further study.

It is difficult to explain the minor significant statistically clusters. While, in this study, there are many minor statistically significant clusters that became significant clusters in the following year or subsequent years while some significant clusters became minor significant clusters conversely. This transformation gives clue to us that the minor statistically significant clusters may be in sub-cluster aggregation state, which also need to be paid attention to, especially for those clusters which had smaller P values (but $P> 0.05$) (Recuenco et al., 2007).

Because surveillance data will be updated year by year, using purely spatial scan statistics to analyze the gradually-increased surveillance data will affect the reliability of the results. Besides, it is very difficult to choose a suitable time span in comprehensive data analysis. If time span is too short, it may not detect the weaker clusters, while if the time span is too long, it may detect the recent clusters ineffectively. Thus, this study adopted space-time permutation scan statistics to analyze the accumulated data from 2005 to 2008, showed that there were some similarities, but differences still existed.

The incidence of syphilis is closely associated with the local social-demographic factors. By retrospective time and/or space scan analysis, we have found the regional and temporal cluster of syphilis, which would direct the further investigation. Finding the factors that attribute to the clusters and taking the intervention measures will benefit the syphilis reduction. The prospectively space-time permutation scan statistics can detect suspicious clusters earlier, which will be more meaningful to prevention on primary and secondary syphilis via public health aspect. It may promote public health officers to conduct investigations, e.g., to find out whether there are any clusters of high risk behavior (gathering parties among men who have sex with men, group drug absorption, etc) and adopt timely and suitable activities. In addition, it will encourage government financial input, which will greatly support the intervention program. In this study, five cluster alarm signals were detected by the prospective space-time permutation scan statistics. It proved the adaptability of applying the method to explore the disease outbreak in primary and secondary syphilis. However, the number of primary and secondary syphilis cases in an individual district was very small in this study, which might cause high variability in rates and introduce errors into calculations. It would be more efficient if more cases were involved, e.g., including all the common sexually transmitted diseases. In fact, only syphilis and gonorrhea were involved in the daily real-time surveillance system in Shenzhen, other sexually transmitted diseases were calculated by weeks. Thus, it called for the real-time surveillance system for common sexually transmitted diseases if we want to make an efficient prediction. Besides, as sexual transmission has been the main transmitted route of HIV infection and syphilis infection will promote HIV infection, early detection and treatment of primary and secondary syphilis will be much more important. Based on the real-time surveillance system, developing early warning system among sexually transmitted diseases, will benefit the control and prevention work.

The syphilis real-time surveillance system was established in 2004 in Shenzhen, thus, the study period was relatively short, involving only four years in this study. The next step is to use the space-time statistics in practical work regularly with the goal of studying the long-term trends of the spatial and temporal clusters of syphilis in Shenzhen.

The epidemic of syphilis could be attributed to varied reasons, including migration of population, number of total population, level of social and economic development, distribution of commercial sex entertainments, number of high risk population, occurrence of unsafe behavior, health resource allocation and service provision. Finding out the factors associated with the spatial and temporal patterns of primary and secondary syphilis cases is essential as it can get a clear picture of the reasons on clusters. However, this study did not collect the related information. This limitation would be considered and improved in the future study.

5. Conclusion

Space-time statistics is an effective method to describe clusters. This study applied the space-time statistics to explore the spatial and temporal patterns of primary and secondary syphilis at neighbourhoods level in Shenzhen. The results showed that the clusters of primary and secondary syphilis cases tend to be distributed towards the regions owing great many migrant workers and entertainment venues, such as Longhua, Cuizu, Huafu, Huangbei and Nanshan street communities, which provided important information on syphilis prevention program as well as the source allocation. The application of prospective space-time permutation scan statistics in this study proved its adaptability among primary and secondary syphilis, and it could detect some risk factors. Moreover, if adding other sexually transmitted disease, e.g., gonorrhea, in the prospective space-time permutation scan statistics, the test would be more effective and the method would produce early warning signals easily. Finally, it would provide useful information for STD and HIV control and prevention. Its efficiency in visualizing public health problems such as syphilis spread also allows policy-maker to target resources more efficiently. SaTScan software is now powerful tool for analyzing and exploring disease incidence, especially some infectious diseases. Further studies to investigate influential factors related to syphilis epidemic in more detail could provide more information to inform risk assessments and control strategies.

6. Acknowledgment

We are grateful to Prof. Liu Xiaoli for technical guidance, Dr. Lan Lina, Dr. Pan Peng, Dr. Zhang Chunlai, Dr. Wen Lizhang for collecting data, Dr. Luo Zhenzhou for entering data on the computers. This work was supported by a grant from Shenzhen Municipal Health Bureau for STI Prevention and Control Programme.

7. References

Cai, YM., Zhang, MH., Zhou, H., Hong, FC., Cheng, JQ., Zhang, YJ. & Zhang, D. (2007). Cost-benefit analysis on project for syphilis prevention of mother-to-child transmission. *Chinese Journal of Public Health*, Vol.23, No. (September 2007), pp. 1062-1063.

Chen, ZQ., Zhang, GC., Gong, XD., Lin, C., Gao, X., Liang, GJ., Yue, XL. Chen, XH. & Cohen, MS. (2007). Syphilis in China: results of a national surveillance programme. *Lancet*, Vol.369, No.13, (January 2007), pp. 132-138.

Cheng, JQ., Zhou, H., Hong, FC., Zhang, D., Zhang, YJ., Pan, P. & Cai, YM. (2007). Syphilis screening and intervention in 500,000 pregnant women in Shenzhen, the People's Republic of China. *Sex Transm Infect*, Vol.83, No.5 (August 2007), pp. 347-350.

Coleman, M., Coleman, M., Mabuza, AM., Kok, G., Coetzee, M. & Durrheim, DN. (2009). Using the SaTScan method to detect local malaria clusters for guiding malaria control programmes. *Malar J*, Vol.8, No. (April 2009), pp. 68.

Feng, TJ., Liu, XL., Cai, YM., Pan, P., Hong, FC., Jiang, WN., Zhou, H. & Chen, XS. (2008). Prevalence of syphilis and human immunodeficiency virus infections among men who have sex with men in Shenzhen, China: 2005 to 2007. *Sex Transm Dis*, Vol.35, No.12 (December 2008), pp. 1022-1024.

Grady, SC. & Enander, H. (2009). Geographic analysis of low birthweight and infant mortality in Michigan using automated zoning methodology. *Int J Health Geogr*, Vol.8 No. (February 2009), pp. 10.

Green, C., Hoppa, RD., Young, TK. & Blanchard JF. (2003). Geographic analysis of diabetes prevalence in an urban area. *Soc Sci Med*, Vol.57, No.3 (August 2003), pp. 551-560.

Haque, U., Huda, M., Hossain, A., Ahmed, SM., Moniruzzaman, M. & Haque, R. (2009). Spatial malaria epidemiology in Bangladeshi highlands. *Malar J*, Vol.8, No. (August 2009), pp. 185.

Hong, FC., Feng, TJ., Cai, YM., Wen, LZ., Pan, P., Lan, LN., Zhou, H., Liu, XL, , Lin, SP., Chen, G. & Chen, XS. (2009a). Burden of syphilis infections in Shenzhen, China: a preliminary estimation. *Int J STD AIDS*, Vol.20, No.2 (February 2009), pp. 115-118.

Hong, FC., Zhou, H., Cai, YM., Pan, P., Feng, TJ., Liu, XL. & Chen, XS. (2009b). Prevalence of syphilis and HIV infections among men who have sex with men from different settings in Shenzhen, China: implications for HIV/STD surveillance. *Sex Transm Infect*, Vol.85, No.1 (February 2009), pp. 42-44.

Hong, FC., Liu, JB., Feng, TJ., Liu, XL., Pan, P., Zhou, H., Cai, YM., Ling, L., Huang, XM., Zhang, D., Zhang, YJ. & Zeegers, MP. (2010). Congenital syphilis: an economic evaluation of a prevention program in China. *Sex Transm Dis*, Vol.37, No.1 (January 2010), pp. 26-31.

Jackson, MC., Huang, L., Luo, J., Hachey, M. & Feuer, E. (2009). Comparison of tests for spatial heterogeneity on data with global clustering patterns and outliers. *Int J Health Geogr*, Vol.8, No. (October 2009), pp. 55.

Kulldorff, M., Athas, WF., Feurer, EJ., Miller, BA. & Key, CR. (1998). Evaluating cluster alarms: a space-time scan statistic and brain cancer in Los Alamos, New Mexico. *Am J Public Health*, Vol.88, No.9 (September 1998), pp. 1377-1380.

Kulldorff, M., Heffernan, R., Hartman, J., Assuncao, R. & Mostashari F. (2005). A space-time permutation scan statistic for disease outbreak detection. *PLoS Med*, No.3 (March 2005), Vol.2, pp. 59.

Meliker, JR., Jacquez, GM., Goovaerts, P., Copeland, G. & Yassine, M. (2009). Spatial cluster analysis of early stage breast cancer: a method for public health practice using cancer registry data. *Cancer Causes Control*, Vol.20, No.7 (September 2009), pp. 1061-1069.

National Center for STD cotnrol, CDC, China. (2010). National epidemic report of syphilis and gonorrhea in 2009. *STD Bulletin*, Vol.1, pp. 1-7.

Newell, J., Senkoro, K., Mosha, F., Grosskurth, H., Nicoll, A., Barongo, L., Borgdorff, M., Klokke, A., Changalucha, J. & Killewo, J. (1993). A population-based study of syphilis and sexually transmitted disease syndromes in north-western Tanzania. 2. Risk factors and health seeking behaviour. *Genitourin Med*, Vol.69, No.6, (December 1993), pp. 421–426.

Recuenco, S., Eidson, M., Kulldorff, M., Johnson, G. & Cherry B. (2007). Spatial and temporal patterns of enzootic raccoon rabies adjusted for multiple covariates. *Int J Health Geogr*, Vol.6, No. (April 2007), pp. 14

Scott, KM., Abhinav, K., Stanton, BR., Johnston, C., Turner, MR., Ampong, MA., Sakel, M., Orrell, RW., Howard, R., Shaw, CE., Leigh, PN. & Al-Chalabi, A. (2009). Geographical clustering of amyotrophic lateral sclerosis in South-East England: a population study. *Neuroepidemiology*, Vol.32, No.2, (February 2009), pp. 81-88.

Stelling, J., Yih, WK., Galas, M., Kulldorff, M., Pichel, M., Terragno, R., Tuduri, E., Espetxe, S., Binsztein, N., O'Brien, TF. & Platt, R. (2009). Automated use of WHONET and SaTScan to detect outbreaks of Shigella spp. using antimicrobial resistance phenotypes. *Epidemiol Infect*, Vol.138, No.6, (Jun 2010), pp. 873-883.

Wallenstein S. (1980). A test for detection of clustering over time. *Am J Epidemiol* , Vol.111, No.3 (March 1980), pp. 367-372.

World Health Organization, Department of Reproductive Health and Research. (2007). The global elimination of congenital syphilis: rationale and strategy for action.

Part 3

Syphilis – Laboratorial Diagnosis

6

Laboratorial Diagnosis of Syphilis

Neuza Satomi Sato
Center of Immunology, Institute Adolfo Lutz
São Paulo, SP
Brazil

1. Introduction

Syphilis is a curable sexually transmitted infection caused by the bacterium *Treponema pallidum*; the infection can also be passed from mother to her fetus during pregnancy.

Diagnosis of syphilis is based on clinical evaluation, detection of the causative organism, and confirmation of the disease by serodiagnosis. *T. pallidum* cannot be cultured in the laboratory, but can be identified in lesions using dark-field or fluorescence microscopy or by molecular techniques. Most infected individuals have no symptoms or have transient lesions and therefore a serological test must be used to screen for infection.

2. Serological tests

Serology is still the most reliable method for laboratory diagnosis of syphilis, regardless of the stage of infection. Serologic test are divided into nontreponemal and treponemal tests, neither alone is sufficient for diagnosis. Conventional serologic diagnosis used a two step approach, of first screening with nontreponemal method, and then using a confirmatory test that uses treponemal antigens based methods to confirm a positive screening test result. Nontreponemal test are usefull also to monitoring treatment response.

The first serologic test for syphilis was the Wassermann test developed in 1906. It was a complement fixation test and the antigen used was an extract of liver from newborn who had died of congenital syphilis. Landsteiner demonstrated that other tissues, such as beef heart extracted in alcohol, could be used equally well as antigens. Cholesterol and lecithin were added to increase the sensitivity of antigens. In 1922, Kahn introduced a flocculation test without complement that could be read macroscopically in a few hours. In 1941, Pangborn isolated from the beef heart the active antigenic component cardiolipin. The pure phospholipid cardiolipin combined with lecithin and cholesterol could be standardized chemically and serologically, ensuring greater reproducibility of test results both within and between laboratories. In 1946, Harris, Rosenberg and Riedel developed the Veneral Disease Research Laboratory (VDRL) and the Rapid Plasma regain (RPR) was developed in 1957, both are still in use currently. The addition of choline chloride and EDTA to the VDRL antigen enhanced the reactivity of the test and stabilized the antigen suspension (Larsen et al., 1995).

The *T. pallidum* was identified in 1905, and the first test identifying treponemal antibodies was developed in 1949 by Nelson and Meyer. The *T. pallidum* immobilization test (TPI) uses *T.pallidum* (Nichols strain) grown in rabbit testes as the antigen and is based on the ability of patient's antibody and complement to immobilize living treponemes, as observed by dark-field microscopy. The fluorescent treponemal antibody (FTA) test was developed in 1957, which was later improved by the absorption procedure (FTA-ABS) in 1964 (Larsen et al., 1995).

2.1 Non-treponemal tests

The most common nontreponemal screening tests include the Veneral Disease Research Laboratory (VDRL) and the Rapid Plasma Reagin (RPR) which detect IgM and IgG antibodies against cardiolipin that is present in the sera of patients with syphilis.

The VDRL test is a slide microfloculation test. The antigen, which is an alcohol solution containing 0.03% cardiolipin, 0.21% lecithin, and 0.9% cholesterol, is suspended in a buffered saline solution. When combined with antibodies, it forms flocculates that are visible using microscope´s low magnification (Larsen et al., 1995).

The RPR is a modification of VDRL test, the antigen for RPR contain choline chloride (to eliminate the inactivation of tested serum), ethylenediaminotetraacetic acid - EDTA (to enhance the stability of the suspension), and charcoal particle for visualization of the suspension. This macroscopic flocculation test is done on plastic cards having multiple 18-mm circles onto which serum and modified VDRL antigen are placed and gently rotated. In the presence of antibodies a flocculation reaction takes place, and the charcoal particles are entrapped in the antigen-antibody aggregates, causing visible agglutination.

The mean sensitivities of the VDRL during primary syphilis, secondary, latent and late latent are 78%, 100%, 95% and 71%, respectively; while sensitivities of RPR are 86%, 100%, 98% and 73%. The mean specificities of both tests are 98% (Larsen et al., 1995).

These tests are widely available, relatively inexpensive and important for monitoring treatment. Only VDRL is the test of choice for examination of cerebrospinal fluid (CSF) in suspected neurosyphilis.

Limitation of the nontreponemal serologic tests include: lack of sensitivity in early primary and late latent syphilis, the possibility of prozone reaction or false positive results (Larsen et al., 1995).

A prozone reaction occurs when antibody is in excess and it is occasionally demonstrated in the nontreponemal serologic tests. Prozone reactions occur in 1 to 2% of patients with secondary syphilis (Jurado et al., 1993).

False positive reactions are associated with increased age, pregnancy, drug addition, malignancy, and auto-imune diseases, such as lupus erythematosus or rheumatoid arthritis, as well as with viral (hepatitis, infectious mononucleosis, viral pneumonia, measles and others), protozoal (malaria) or mycoplasma infection (Hook & Marra, 1992; Larsen et al., 1995).

Nontreponemal test results must be interpreted according to the stage of syphilis disease. Also, the interpretation of these results depends on the population being tested. The predicitive value of the nontreponemal tests is increased when combined with a reactive treponemal tests (Larsen et al., 1995).

2.2 Treponemal tests

Treponemal tests which are based in antigens derived from *T.pallidum*, allow detection of specific anti-treponemal antibodies. These tests have higher sensitivity and specificity than nontreponemal and were used as confirmatory tests for syphilis after a reactive nontreponemal on screening.

Treponemal tests include the fluorescent treponemal antibody-absorbed test (FTA-ABS), *Treponema pallidum* hemaglutination assay (TPHA), *Treponema pallidum* particle agglutination (TPPA) and enzyme immunoassay (EIA).

Treponemal tests may remain reactive for years with or without treatment. Therefore, these tests should not be used to evaluate response to therapy, relapse or re-infection in previously treated patients. Also, it do not differentiate veneral syphilis from endemic syphilis (yaw and pinta). However, one treponemal IgM test, the Captia Syphilis-M EIA showed high sensitivity in primary syphilis(Lefevre et al., 1990) and also useful in monitoring treatment response of early syphilis (McMillan & Young, 2008).

2.2.1 FTA-ABS

The FTA-ABS test is an indirect fluorescent-antibody technique, the antigen used is *T.pallidum* subsp. *pallidum* (Nichols strain). The patient's serum is diluted 1:5 in sorbent (an extract from cultures of the nonpathogenic Reiter treponeme) to remove group treponemal antibodies that are produced in some person in response to nonpathogenic treponemes. The absorbed serum is layered on a microscope slide to which *T.pallidum* has been fixed. If the patient's serum contains antibody, it coats the treponeme. FICT-labeled anti-human immunoglobulin is added and combines with the patient's antibodies resulting in FICT-stained spirochetes that are visible when examined by a fluorescence microscope. The mean sensitivities of the FTA-ABS during primary syphilis and late latent are 84% and 96%, respectively; while the sensitivities during secondary and recent latent syphilis are 100%. The mean specificities are 97%(Larsen et al., 1995). Until recently, FTA-ABS was considered the "gold standard" serological test for laboratorial diagnosis of syphilis.

2.2.2 TPHA and TPPA

Hemagglutination test was developed in the same era as the FTA-ABS test. It is technically simpler test and detects reactive antibody that agglutinates red blood cells sensitized with *T.pallidum* antigen (Rathlev, 1967; Rudolph, 1976; Tomizawa, 1966).

A formalinized, tanned sheep (or turkey) erythrocytes are sensitized with ultrasonicated antigen from *T.pallidum*, Nichols strain. The patient's serum is first mixed with absorbing diluents made from nonpathogenic Reiter treponemes and other absorbents and stabilizers. The reaction is performed in a microtiter plate. Serum containing antibodies reacts with these cells to form a smooth mat of agglutinated cells in the microtiter plate. Unsensitized cells are used as a control for nonspecific reactivity. The mean sensitivities of the TPHA during primary syphilis, latent and late latent are 76%, 97-100% and 94%, respectively; while the sensitivities during secondary is 100%. The mean specificities are 99% (Larsen et al., 1995).

The *T.pallidum* particle agglutination assay (TPPA) uses biologically inert colored gel particles in place of red blood cells and has fewer equivocal reactions than the hemagglutination test, because heterophile reactions are eliminated (Deguchi et al., 1994). The mean sensitivities of the TPPA during primary syphilis, secondary and latent syphilis are 88%, 100% and 98%, respectively, while the mean specificities are 95% (Pope et al., 2000).

2.2.3 EIA

Veldkamp and Visser recognized the potencial for na automated *T.pallidum* enzyme-linked immunosorbent assay in the 1970s (Veldkamp & Visser, 1975). Since then, several EIAs using either native or recombinant *T.pallidum* antigens have been developed and numerous are commercially available. EIA reported in the literature have used different approach to determine sensitivities and specificities. Some studies had used a panel of anti-treponemal positive specimens from patients whose disease stage and treatment status was known and a negative serum from health blood donors. Other studies had evaluated the performance of new test by comparing with results of conventional laboratorial tests used for diagnosis of syphilis. In general, EIA presents higher sensitivity and specificity.

Captia Syphilis G (Trinity Biotech, former Centocor) is an indirect test for detection of treponemal antibodies. This test uses microtitration plates or strips coated with sonicated *T.pallidum* antigen. The reacting human IgG treponemal antibodies are detected by anti-human IgG monoclonal antibodies labeled with biotin and horse radish peroxidase (HRP) labeled streptavidin and revealed by tetramethylbenzidine (TMB) substrate. The sensitivity has ranged from 92.4% to 100% and specificity from 98.2% to 99.3%(Halling et al., 1999; Silletti, 1995; Young et al., 1989; Young et al., 1998). The newer Captia select Syph-G EIA (Trinity Biotech) using anti-human IgG monoclonal antibodies labeled with HRP as a conjugate instead of biotin-streptavidin system had sensitivity and specificity of 99.0% and 98.0%, respectively (Woznicova & Valisova, 2007).

Enzygnost Syphilis (Dade Behring) is a one step competitive EIA with *T.pallidum* Nichols strain detergent extract antigen. *T.pallidum* specific antibodies, IgG and/or IgM contained in the sample and the conjugate (HRP labeled anti-Tp antibodies) compete for the binding sites of *T.pallidum* antigen coated onto wells of microtitration plates. The reaction is revealed with substrate TMB. The intensity of the resultant color is inversely proportional to the concentration of anti-treponemal antibodies in the sample. Enzygnost Syphilis showed sensitivities varying from 98.2% to 100% and specificities from 96.8% to 100% (Cole et al., 2007; Gutierrez et al., 2000; Maidment et al., 1998; Marangoni Antonella et al., 2009; Viriyataveekul et al., 2006).

Bioelisa Syphilis (Biokit) is a competitive assay using *T.pallidum* whole antigen to coat the well of a plate. The treponemal antibodies in the test serum compete with HRP labeled human anti-treponemal antibodies. In this assay, the binding of the conjugate to the specific antigen, determined by measuring the intensity of substrate (TMB) color, is inversely proportional to the amount of specific antibodies in the test sample. Compared with FTA-ABS and TPHA, this assay had sensitivity of 99.5% and specificity of 99.4% (Ebel et al., 1998). Another version of this assay, Bioelisa Syphilis 3.0 (Biokit) is a two step recombinant EIA using recombinant antigen (TpN15 and TpN17) to coat the solid phase and HRP conjugated recombinant antigen for detection of anti-treponemal IgG and IgM. This assay showed sensitivity of 97.4%, and specificity of 100%. However, lower detection rate was observed in samples from patients with untreated primary syphilis (Cole et al., 2007).

ICE Syphilis (Murex) is a two step recombinant sandwich EIA using three *T. pallidum* recombinant antigen (TpN15, TpN17 and TpN47) coated onto the wells of microtiter plate strips; the wells are also coated with anti-human immunoglobulin G (IgG) and M (IgM). If the antibodies to *T.pallidum* are present in the specimens (serum or plasma) they are captured by the antigen on the plate. In addition, a proportion of a total IgG and IgM of tested specimens are captured by the anti-human antibodies. The anti-treponemal components of the captured antibodies is detected by recombinant antigens (TpN15, TpN17 and TpN47) labeled with HRP. The intensity of the enzyme substrate TMB color is proportional to the concentration of antibodies reacting with recombinant *T.pallidum* antigens. The range of sensitivity and specificity for the ICE Syphilis assay were 98.2% to 100% and 99.2% to 100%, respectively (Cole et al., 2007; Lam et al., 2010; Viriyataveekul et al., 2006; Young et al., 1998). Other studies for evaluation of ICE Syphilis (Murex) as a screening test for syphilis, the sensitivity in primary syphilis were 84% (48/50) (Manavi & McMillan, 2007) and 77.2% (61/79)(Young et al., 2009).

Trep-Chek (Phoenix) is an indirect test for detection of anti-treponemal antibodies. The microplates wells is coated with specific recombinant treponemal antigens. Anti-treponemal antibodies present in the serum samples binds to the immobilized antigens. Anti-human IgG antibodies labeled with HRP and substrate TMB are used to detect specific anti-treponemal antibodies present in the patient´s samples. when compared with results of convencional serological tests, the sensitivity and specificity for Trep-chek was 85.3% and 95.6%, respectively (Tsang et al., 2007); other study found sensitivity of 98.9% and specificity of 95.6% in comparison with results of FTA-ABS (Binnicker et al., 2011).

Trep-Sure (Phoenix) is a two step recombinant sandwich EIA for detection of anti-treponemal antibodies IgG and IgM. This assay uses specific recombinant treponemal antigens immobilized on the microplate wells. Anti-treponemal antibodies from patient´s samples bind to the immobilized antigen, which is detected with HRP conjugated treponemal antigens and substrate TMB. Trep-Sure had sensitivity and specificity of 98.9% and 94.3%, respectively (Binnicker et al., 2011).

Captia Syphilis M (Trinity, former Centocor) is a capture ELISA using a microtitration plates coated with anti-human μ chain specific antibodies, which bind IgM present in serum. A tracer complex is used to detect anti-treponemal specific IgM antibody captured on the plate. The tracer complex consisted of *T. pallidum* antigens, a biotinylated antiaxial filament monoclonal IgM antibody, and streptavidin conjugated with horseradish peroxidase. The enzyme substrate TMB yields a colored product and the intensity of the color is proporcional to the concentration of antibodies (Lefevre et al., 1990); newer version of this assay employ a HRP conjugated recombinant antigen instead of the tracer complex (Rotty et al., 2010). This EIA was specifically designed for diagnosis of congenital syphilis, but may be applied for detection of primary infection. The sensitivity was 94% for primary syphilis, 85% for secondary, and 82% for early latent syphilis (Lefevre et al., 1990). This IgM capture EIA is also useful for monitoring treatment response in early syphilis (McMillan & Young, 2008; Rotty et al., 2010).

Schmidt et al performed a comparative evaluation of different EIAs for determination of antibodies against *T.pallidum* in patients with primary syphilis by testing 52 sera, all negative in TPHA. The sensitivity for Captia Syphilis M was 86.5% (45/52) and other assays for detection of IgG and IgM, such as ICE Syphilis (Murex), Enzygnost Syphilis (Berhing) and Bioelisa Syphilis (Biokit) showed sensitivities of 75.0% (39/52), 69.2% (36/52) and 67.3 (24/41), respectively (Schmidt et al., 2000).

2.2.4 Immunochemoluminescence assay (CIA) and multiplex flow immunoassay (MFI)

In addition to EIA, new treponemal assay based on CIA or MFI technology are available with the advantage of automation facilities, higher testing throughput and the objective interpretation.

The LIAISON Treponema screen (Diasorin) is a one-step sandwich chemiluminescence immunoassay (LIAISON CLIA) that measures total anti-treponemal antibody (IgG and IgM). A recombinant treponemal antigen (TpN17) is coated onto paramagnetic microparticles and patient's serum (or plasma) are added along with an isoluminol-antigen conjugate. The same antigen TpN17 is component of conjugate. Specific anti-treponemal antibodies present in the specimen will be captured to the antigen on the paramagnetic particle and bind to the antigen conjugate in a sandwich manner. After incubation, unbound material is removed with a wash cycle. Starter reagents are added and a light signal is produced from a flash chemiluminescence reaction if anti-treponemal antibodies are present. The light signal is measured by a photomultipler as Relative Light Units (RLU), and the results are reported as an index value.

A retrospective study performed by Marangoni et al analyzed a panel of 2,494 blood donor sera, 131 clinically and serologically characterized syphilitic sera and 96 samples obtained from subjects with potentially interfering diseases or conditions (including Lyme disease, mononucleosis, rheumatoid factor positive and *T.denticola* positive). Also, 1,800 unselected samples submitted for routine screening for syphilis was included in this study. LIAISON sensitivity was 99.2%, which was higher than EIA (95.4%) or TPHA (94.7%) especially when primary syphilis samples were tested. Only Western Blot had 100% sensitivity. In this study LIAISON missed detection of a sample from treated latent syphilis patient. Specificity was 99.9% for all treponemal tests. From 96 sera obtained from patient suffering from potentially cross-reactive conditions, no serum gave a positive result by LIAISON (Marangoni et al., 2005). However, another study for evaluation of LIAISON test found lower sensitivity of 94.1% (48/51), in primary and secondary syphilis (Knight et al., 2007).

The Abbott ARCHITECT Syphilis TP assay is a two-step sandwich chemiluminescent microparticle immunoassay (CMIA) for the qualitative detection of antibody to *Treponema pallidum* in human serum or plasma based on recombinant antigens TpN15, TpN17 and TpN47. Antibody present in the sample binds to *T.pallidum* recombinant antigen coated paramagnetic particles. After wash step, murine anti-human-IgG/anti-human-IgM acridinium-labelled conjugate is added. Following a further wash step, pre-trigger solution (hydrogen peroxide) and trigger solution (sodium hydroxide) are added. The resulting chemiluminescent reaction is measured in relative light units (RLUs) which are directly proportional to the amount of anti-*T.pallidum* present in the sample. The Architect Syphilis was highly sensitive in detecting primary syphilis(97.5%) and had specificity of 99.1% (Young et al., 2009). In another evaluation, this assay presented 100% sensitivity (121/121) and specificity (500/500) and good performance on reproducibility, with intra-assay coefficient variation lower than 4% (Yoshioka et al., 2007).

Recently, Wellinghausen & Dietenberger evaluated two automated CIA, the LIAISON Treponema Screen and the ARCHITECT Syphilis TP in comparison to the TPPA test for laboratory diagnosis of syphilis. A prospective study was performed using 577 sera submitted for diagnosis of syphilis and 42 stored sera from patients with syphilis infection diagnosed by clinic and serology. Sensitivity was 100% for all three tests, and specificity were 100%, 99,8% and 99,6% respectively for LIAISON, ARCHTECT and TPPA (Wellinghausen & Dietenberger, 2011).

Bio-Rad BioPlex 2200 Syphilis Multiplex Flow Immunoassay (MFI) was evaluated for the detection of anti-treponemal antibodies, IgM and IgG. The principle of MFI technology is based on cytometric beads array.

The BioPlex Syphilis IgG kit uses three different populations of microspheres coated with recombinant proteins from *T.pallidum* (15 kDa, 17 kDa and 47 kDa). The patient's specimens is added to a reaction vessel containing bead reagent and sample diluents and incubated at 37°C. Antibody present in the sample binds to *T.pallidum* recombinant antigen coated beads. After wash step, a phycoerytrin-conjugated reporter antibody is added. After second incubation and washing step, the beads are read by a flow-based detector which quantitates each analyte and compares it to a pre-established calibration curve. The data are initially calculated as relative fluorescence intensity and then converted to a fluorescence ratio (FR) using an internal standard bead. The FR is compared to an assay specific calibration curve to determine the analyte concentration in antibody index (AI) units, where AI is higher than 1.0 for positive samples and lower than 1.0 for negative one.

The kits for IgM uses two different beads sets individually coated with recombinant proteins associated with *T.pallidum* (17 and 47 kDa).

In a prospective analysis of 1008 serum samples submitted for serologic testing for syphilis, the BioPlex IgG MFI assay demonstrated sensitivity of 98.7% (77/78) and specificity of 99.4% (916/930) in comparison with EIA assay. For anti-treponemal IgM antibody detection, BioPlex IgM MFI assay showed 80% (4/5) sensitivity and 97.9% (652/666) specificity, when compared to the Trep-Chek IgM EIA (Phoenix-Biotech). BioPlex syphilis MFI assay allow for a fully automated random-accesses platform that provides fast (1.7h for 100 samples) and high throughput (800 samples per 9 hours) analysis of the syphilis serologic response (Gomez et al., 2010).

2.2.5 Westen Blot (WB) and Immuno-blot

Immunoblotting allows for the detection of antibodies to individual proteins. In the Treponemal Western blot (Tp-WB), solubilized *T.pallidum* proteins are separated by gel electrophoresis according to their molecular size. The separated proteins are then transferred onto a nitrocellulose membrane which is dried and cut into strips. After incubating the strips with patient's serum, antigen-antibody complexes are visualized by adding enzyme-conjugated anti-human globulin followed by substrate, which causes a color reaction. It is generally agreed that detection of antibodies to immunodeterminants with molecular masses of 15, 17, 44.5 and 47kDa (TpN15, TpN17, TpN44.5 and TpN47) are diagnostic for acquired syphilis.

	Reference	Sensitivity		Specificity	
1.	Byrne et al, 1992	93.8 %	(45/48)	100%	(25/25)
2.	Young et al, 1994	99.1 %	(113/114)	88.2%	(15/17)
3.	George et al, 1998	94.3%	(117/124)	98.0%	(347/354)
4.	Marangoni et al, 1999	100%	(35/35)	100%	(45/45)
5.	Backhouse et al, 2001	100%	(98/98)	100%	(128/128)
6.	Lemos et al, 2006	100%	(122/122)	99.5%	(383/385)
7.	Welch et al, 2010	98.2%	(65/66)	100%	(134/134)
8.	Lam et al, 2010	65.2%	(88/135)	100%	(43/43)
9.	Sato et al, 2004	95.1 %	(58/61)	94.7%	(72/76)
10.	Welch et al, 2010	95.5%	(63/66)	97.8%	(131/134)
11.	Binnicker et al, 2011	93.8%	(91/97)	98.5%	(203/206)
12.	Ebel et al, 2000	99.6%	(462/464)	99.5%	(369/371)
13.	Hagedorn et al, 2002	100%	(219/219)	99.3%	(286/288)
14.	Lam et al, 2010	94.1%	(127/135)	100%	(43/43)

Table 1. Performance of WB (1 - 8, native antigen) and Dot-Blot (9 – 14, recombinant antigen) tests for serological diagnosis of syphilis.

The Tp-WB showed a high sensitivity in both, treated and untreated infection (Young et al., 1994). One study found that the 17 kDa antigen have the best combined attributes of sensitivity and specificity for diagnostic of syphilis (George et al., 1998). Another study found that a more sensitive and specific criterion for the WB would be the reactivity with the antigen of 15kDa and other two of the three major antigens, TpN47, TpN44.5 and TpN17. The criterion was based on the analysis of reactivity for individual antigenic determinant where only the antigen of TpN15 had 100% sensitivity and specificity. For other three antigens the sensitivities were 100%, 100%, 96% and the specificities were 20%, 96%, 100%, respectively for of TpN47, TpN44.5 and TpN17 (Backhouse & Nesteroff, 2001).

Lemos et al (2006) evaluated the association of clinical phases of syphilis with the reactivity of individual antigenic determinants. The reaction with TpN47 was present in all phases of syphilis, with higher intensity in primary and early syphilis than in late latent and tertiary syphilis. The reaction to TpN17 was observed in samples from patients with early syphilis (primary, secondary and early latent). Except to patients with primary syphilis, samples from patients with any of the other clinical forms of syphilis showed reactivity against TpN15. In tertiary syphilis, the reactivity of TpN15 showed higher intensity than TpN47 (de Lemos et al., 2007).

Recently, a commercially available treponemal WB kit has been evaluated for its use as confirmatory test for the serological diagnosis of syphilis (Lam et al., 2010; Welch & Litwin, 2010). The TWB (MarDx Diagnostics, CA, USA) is a Western Blot assay and uses three native antigens (15.5, 17 and 47 kDa) to detect IgG antitreponemal antibody.

One study was carried with 200 serum samples collected for routine laboratorial diagnosis of syphilis, which were separated according to the results of classical syphilis tests, RPR and FTA-ABS. The TWB - MarDx assay showed a sensitivity of 98.2%, specificity of 100% and overall agreement of 99.4% (Lam et al., 2010; Welch & Litwin, 2010). Another study was performed with 173 serum samples from patients in different clinical stage, including primary syphilis (39), secondary (20), early latent (18), latent of unknown duration (58) and normal health subjets (43). The overall sensitivity was as low as 65.2%. The highest sensitivity of 90% was found in secondary stage and the lowest was 50% in the latent stage of unknown duration, whereas in primary and early latent stages the sensitivity was around 72%. This assay presented 38 samples (28.1%) with indeterminate results (Lam et al., 2010; Welch & Litwin, 2010).

Based on published data, Tp-WB showed specificity from 88 - 100% and sensitivity ranging from 94-100%, except for one study that found sensitivity of 65.2% for TWB kit. Overall, these native antigen based Tp-WB assay is a useful additional confirmatory test for syphilis.

A blot assay using recombinant antigens instead of fractionates native proteins had been described (Sato et al., 2004) and some are also commercially available, including Treponema Virablot IgG (Viramed Biotech) (Binnicker et al., 2011; Welch & Litwin, 2010) and INNO-LIA (Immunogenetics, Belgium) (Ebel et al., 2000).

The immune-slot-blot assay is an "in house" technique prepared with three recombinant antigen rTp47, rTp17 and rTp15 immobilized on nitrocellulose strip. It was analyzed 137 serum samples from patients with a clinical and laboratory diagnosis of syphilis (61), from healthy blood donors (50), individuals with sexually transmitted disease other than syphilis (3), and from individuals with other spirochetal diseases such as Lyme disease (20) and leptospirosis (3). The sensitivity was 95.1% (58/61) and specificity was 94.7% (72/76) (Sato et al., 2004).

The Treponema Virablot IgG (Viramed Biotech) is composed with Tp47, Tp44.5, Tp17 and Tp15 and it was evaluated with serum samples previously analyzed with classical serological tests for diagnosis of syphilis. In comparison with results of RPR, FTA-ABS and TPPA, the sensibility was 95.5% and the specificity was 97.8% (Welch, 2010). Similar results was found by Binnicker et al, the sensibility and specificity were 93.8% and 98.5%, respectively, when compared with FTA-ABS (Binnicker et al., 2011).

The INNO-LIA Syphilis test (Innogenetics) is a line immunoassay utilizing three recombinant antigens of *T.pallidum* (TpN 47, TpN17 and TpN15) and one synthetic peptide derived from TpN44.5 (TmpA), which coated as discrete lines on nylon.

This assay was initially validated by using a large number of sera (835) from a clinical laboratory and the overall sensitivity and specificity were calculated with reference to consensus diagnostic assay results. The INNO-LIA Syphilis test had sensitivity of 99.6% and specificity of 99.5% (Ebel et al., 2000). These results were confirmed by another evaluation of the assay using 507 serum samples, the sensitivity and specificity were 100% and 99.3%, respectively (Hagedorn et al., 2002). Recently, the test was analyzed with 135 serum samples from patients in different clinical stages of syphilis. A lower sensitivity of 94.1% was determined in this group. The sensitivity were 92.3%, 100%, 94.4% and 94.1%, respectively for primary, secondary, early latent and latent of unknown duration clinical stages of syphilis (Lam et al., 2010). The INNO-LIA syphilis test provides highly reliable results and can be considered to be a valid alternative confirmatory for serological tests for syphilis.

2.2.6 Treponema specific rapid diagnostic test (point of care - POC)

A number of simple, point-of-care (POC) treponema specific rapid diagnostic tests are also commercially available. Most rapid tests detect IgM, IgG and IgA antibodies and involve immunochromatographic strips in which one or multiple *T.pallidum* recombinant antigens are applied to nitrocellulose strips as a capture reagent. Antibodies in the specimen bound at antigen site on the strip and are revealed with dye bound anti-immunoglobulin or dye bound antigen and a positive reaction appears as a colored line.

Most of these tests can be used with whole blood from a finger prick as well as serum or plasma. The results can be read visually in less than 30 minutes, these rapid tests are simple to perform, require minimal equipment and training. It is suitable for use in primary healthcare settings, and also it can be performed in the field at point of care.

Overall, rapid tests are highly sensitive and specific. The World Health Organization compared the performance of 8 rapid tests to a combined reference standart TPHA/TPPA, reporting sensitivities of 84.5%-97.7% and specificities of 92.8% - 98% (Herring et al., 2006). A lower sensitivity was found for a whole blood in comparison with serum or plasma. Additionally, the sensitivity was lower in the field conditions than in assay performed in the laboratory (Benzaken et al., 2008; Mabey et al., 2006a; Mishra et al., 2010).

Determine Syphilis TP (Abbott) has recombinant antigen TpN47 immobilized on nitrocellulose strips and use 50uL of sample, either whole blood, serum or plasma and results can be read in 5 to 20 minutes. For serum or plasma specimens, sensitivity range were 93.7 to 99.2% and specificity 92.4 to 100% (Diaz et al., 2004; Herring et al., 2006; Mabey et al., 2006a; Mabey et al., 2006b; Oshiro et al., 1999; Sato et al., 2003). For whole blood sample, the sensitivity ranged from 85,9% to 95.0%, and specificity was higher than 97.7% (Gianino et al., 2007; Mabey et al., 2006a; Siedner et al., 2004; Tinajeros et al., 2006) when performed in the reference laboratory. Lower sensitivity of 75.6% was found when the assay was performed at local clinic (Li et al., 2009; Mabey et al., 2006a).

SD BioLine Syphilis 3.0 ICS (Standard Diagnostics, Korea) use three recombinant antigens TpN15, TpN17 and TpN47 to capture specific antibodies. The assay is performed with 20 uL of whole blood or 10 uL of serum or plasma, and results can be read in 5 to 20 minutes.

For serum samples, overall sensitivities were 94.2 -95.0% and specificities 94.9% - 97.8%(Herring et al., 2006; Mabey et al., 2006a). However, for whole blood samples, this rapid test showed better sensitivities for assay performed in the laboratory when compared with local clinic testing. These differences were observed in the results obtained at three countries (Tanzania, Brazil and China), according to the study published by Mabey et al. Sensitivities ranged from 90.2% to 95.5% and 85.7% to 88.2%, respectively for laboratory and local clinic testing. Specifities were 95.5% to 99.4% and 98.8% to 99.6%, respectively (Mabey et al., 2006a). Montoya et al found similar results; sensitivities were 96.3% and 86.0%, respectively for laboratory and healthy facility testing, while specificity showed no difference, 96.8% and 96.4% (Herring et al., 2006; Mabey et al., 2006a; Montoya et al., 2006).

Visitec Syphilis (Omega Diagnostics, Scotland UK) uses two recombinant antigens TpN17 and TpN47 to capture specific antibodies. The assay is performed with 50 uL of whole blood or 25 uL of serum or plasma, and results can be read in 15 minutes.

For serum samples, sensitivities were 84.2% to 98.2% and specificities 98.0% to 99.1% (Herring et al., 2006; Mabey et al., 2006a). For whole blood samples, sensitivities were 77.9% to 98.2% and 72.7% to 96.1% respectively for laboratory and local clinic testing, while overall specificities were around 99% for both settings (Herring et al., 2006; Mabey et al., 2006a).

A finger prick blood samples were tested with Visitec Syphilis to assess the performance of this rapid test to o detect syphilis in field evaluation of high risk populations. Visitec Syphilis test had identified 79% (30/38) of active syphilis cases (Benzaken et al., 2008).

Qualpro Syphicheck-WB rapid syphilis test (Qualpro Diagnostic, India) use two recombinant antigens TpN17 and TpN47 to capture specific antibodies. The assay is performed with 50 uL of whole blood or 25 uL of serum or plasma, and results can be read in 15 minutes.

For serum samples, sensitivities were 84.5% to 95.3% and specificities 93.7 to 98.9% (Herring et al., 2006; Mabey et al., 2006a). For whole blood samples, sensitivities were 70.8% to 97.6% and 64.0% to 84.3% respectively for laboratory and local clinic testing, while overall specificities were around 99% for both settings (Herring et al., 2006; Mabey et al., 2006a).

The Syphcheck-WB test using finger prick whole blood was evaluated for detection of active syphilis among female sex workers in Bangalore, India. Compared with the reference RPR and TPHA, the sensitivity and specificity of the POC syphilis were 70.8% and 97.8%, respectively (Mishra et al., 2010).

Besides its lower sensitivity, this study revealed that the use of POC screening conferred an advantage over offsite RPR testing among hard-to-reach populations, who may not return for their test results and follow-up treatment. The proportion of women with active syphilis who were appropriately treated rose from 44.8% to 68.3% (p=0.003) with the use of POC syphilis screening (Mishra et al., 2010).

The limitation of rapid syphilis tests is that they cannot distinguish active and treated syphilis; positive results need confirmation with quantitative nontreponemal testing to determine recent infection and response to therapy.

New approach based POC tests has been described and it may be promissory to overcome the limitations of rapid tests currently available.

Recently, a novel dual POC syphilis test had been developed for simultaneous detection of nontreponemal and treponemal antibodies in patients with syphilis. Compared with RPR, the concordance of the dual non-treponemal line was 98.4% and the nonreactive concordance was 98.6%. Compared to the TPPA assay, the reactive and nonreactive concordances of the treponemal line were 96.5% and 95.5%, respectively (Castro et al., 2010).
The test for detection of *T. pallidum* specific IgM antibody named colloidal gold immunochromatography assay (GICA) had been described by Lin et al. GICA has monoclonal antibody to the human μ chain-specific IgM immobilized on nitrocellulose strips to capture the patient treponemal-specific IgM which is revealed by the colloidal gold conjugated recombinant antigens, TpN17 and TpN47. The sensitivity and specificity were 98.2% and 99.0% when compared with FTA-IgM (Lin et al., 2011).
These new POC test can be helpful for diagnosing active syphilis disease.

3. Direct detection of *Treponema pallidum*

There are number of methods available for direct detection of intact organisms or *T.pallidum* DNA.

3.1 Darkfield microscopy

The oldest method still remains one of the simplest and most reliable for the direct detection of *T. pallidum*. An experienced microscopist can identify *T.pallidum* from lesions based on the characteristic morphology and motility of the spirochete. This method is suitable when the lesions are moist, and the examination can be done immediately after specimen collection. Exudates and fluids from lesions are examined as a wet mount using dark-field microscopy. During the primary stage, serous fluid from the lesion contains numerous treponemes and, therefore, this approach is particularly useful in patients with immunodeficiency or in early syphilis when antibodies are not yet detectable. Success is dependent on a number of factors, including too little or too much fluid on the slide, the presence of refractile elements in the specimen, improper thickness of the slide or cover slip, etc. Treatment with antibiotics may result in a false-negative finding. Therefore, although the demonstration of *T pallidum* is the definitive method of diagnosis, dark-field microscopy has limited sensitivity, and failure to detect *T pallidum* by this test does not rule out syphilis (Larsen S.A. et al., 1990).

3.2 Direct fluorescent antibody test for *T.pallidum* (DFA-TP) in the blood fluids

The direct fluorescent antibody test for *T.pallidum* is easier to perform than dark-field microscopy, it detects antigens and does not require the presence of motile treponemes. DFA-TP test use fluorescein isothiocyanate-labelled anti-*T.pallidum* antibody to identify the organism. However, this test does not differentiate between *T.pallidum* and other pathogenic treponemes causing yaws, endemic syphilis and pinta specific to pathogenic treponemes. The number organisms in the fluid or tissue that can be detected by fluorescent antibody tests is similar to that for darkfiled micoscopy. The sensitivity of these methods is only stightly better than darkfiled microscopy (Larsen S.A. et al., 1990).

3.3 Direct test for *T.pallidum* in tissue sections

Direct fluorescent antibody test for *T.pallidum* using fluorescein isothiocyanate-labelled anti-*T.pallidum* antibody can also be used in tissue section to identify the organism (DFAT-T).

Immunohistochemical (IHC) detection of *T.pallidum* use an unlabeled treponemal antibody and the detection complex based on secondary antibody, enzyme conjugate and insoluble enzyme substrate system for IHC stain. This method can be used in combination with histological staining; the advantage of hematoxylin counterstain is to examine tissue structure simultaneously.

Silver staining, while useful, is nonspecific. Silver nitrate will impregnate a number of different organisms and allows only for identification of the morphology of the organism. tissue artifacts are a potential hazard for misidentification (Larsen S.A. et al., 1990).

3.4 Rabbit Infectivity Test (RIT)

RIT is probably the most sensitive methods for detecting infectious treponeme. Any source of specimen can be used for RIT as long as the material is less than 1 hour old or was flash-frozen immediately after collection and maintained in liquid nitrogen or at temperature of -78°C or bellow.

The RIT remains a research tool of academic interest for detection of virulent organism in clinical specimens because of the need for animal, the very long incubation time after infection (several weeks to months), and variation in rabbit susceptibility to infection (Larsen S.A. et al., 1990).

This technique was also used as a gold standard for measuring the sensitivity of methods such as PCR. The RIT, using susceptible rabbit, has a sensitivity of 10 to 50 organisms, similar to that of DNA PCR (Grimprel et al., 1991; Sanchez et al., 1993).

3.5 Polymerase Chain Reaction (PCR)

A number of PCR based methods have been developed for the detection of *T.pallidum* DNA or RNA in clinical specimens. These assays are based on the detection of various target genes including tmpA (a 45kDa membrane protein Hay, 1990a); bmp, 39-kDa basic membrane protein (Noordhoek et al., 1991); tpp47, a 47kDa membrane immunogen (Burstain et al., 1991); polA, DNA polymerase I (Liu et al., 2001); tmpC, a 35kDa membrane protein (Flasarova et al., 2006) and 16SrRNA (Centurion-Lara et al., 1997).

The first application PCR in clinical samples from patients with syphilis was reported by Hay et al in 1990. They used primers derived from the gene sequence of TmpA and the 4D antigen (and oligomeric protein with multiple forms). The detection limit was 65 organisms. When PCR was used to detect *T.pallidum* DNA in cerebrospinal fluid (CSF) of patients with and without syphilis, sensitivity was 47% and specificity 93% (Hay et al., 1990a; Hay et al., 1990b).

The bmp gene was used as target for nested-PCR described by Noordhoek et al. Initially, a 617-bp (171-788) portion of bmp gene was amplified and used for second PCR to generate the 500 bp (256-762) products, which was detected with ^{32}P-labeled probe of 19 nt (500-519). The detection limit was 1 fg DNA (1 organism). PCR was applied to detect *T.pallidum* DNA in CSF from neurosyphilis patients before and after antibiotic treatment. Prior to treatment, PCR was positive in 71% (5/7) patients with acute symptomatic and 12% (2/16) asymptomatic neurosyphilis. However, they found treponemal DNA in CSF up to 3 year after treatment (Noordhoek et al., 1991).

Brustain et al had used this same bmp gene as target in a multiplex PCR for simultaneous detection of *T.pallidum* and *Haemophilus ducrey* DNA in genital ulcer samples. The nested PCR product was analyzed on a 10% polyacrylamide gel by using ethidium bromide staining. Multiplex nested PCR showed higher sensitivity then serological methods for diagnosis of syphilis in the population studied, from outpatient clinic for sexually transmitted diseases (STDs) in Amsterdan. Sensitivity and specificity were 75% (12/16) and 100% (348/348), respectively (Bruisten et al., 2001).

The ttp47 gene PCR to detect *T.pallidum* DNA in clinical samples was developed by Burstain et al. A 658-bp (648-1305) portion of tpp47 gene was amplified and the PCR products were probed by DNA-DNA hybridization with a 496-bp (713-1208) fragment internal to the amplified DNA. The assay detected approximately 0.01 pg of purified *T. pallidum* DNA, and it was able to detect as low as one to 10 organisms per specimen with high sensitivity. *T. pallidum* DNA was detected in serum, CSF and amniotic fluids from syphilis patients but not in nonsyphilitic controls (Bruisten et al., 2001). The same technique was applied in several clinical materials in order to investigate the potential of PCR in diagnosis of congenital syphilis. The PCR was 100% specific for *T. pallidum* compared with the sensitive rabbit infectivity test (RIT) for all clinical materials tested. Sensitivities for amniotic fluids, CSF and serum were 100%, 60% and 67% respectively (Grimprel et al., 1991).

Kouznetsov et al used nested-PCR to amplify a different portion of ttp47 gene. The 379 bp (357-735) PCR product was used to amplify the 194 bp (391-584) products by nested-PCR; detection was performed by ^{32}P-labeled probe of 19 bp (481-499), and the detection limit was 20 organism (Kouznetsov & Prinz, 2002). The ttp47 gene was detected in 80% (12/15) of peripheral blood mononuclear cells (PBMCs) from patients with syphilis; when serum samples were analyzed the PCR was positive in 83% (5/6) patients with secondary syphilis and in 50% (2/4) patients with early latent syphilis (Kouznetsov et al., 2005).

A smaller fragment of 260 bp (537-776) of tpp47 was targeted in multiplex-PCR (M-PCR). This M-PCR assay with colorimetric detection was devised for the simultaneous amplification of DNA targets from *H. ducreyi, T. pallidum,* and herpes simplex virus (HSV) types 1 and 2. The assay detected from 1 to 10 organisms. In analysis of 298 genital ulcer swabs, M-PCR showed higher sensitivity (91%) when compared with darkfield microscopy (81%), the specificity was 99%(Orle et al., 1996).

The same target (260 bp) was used by Palmer et al to evaluated PCR for diagnosis of early syphilis. DNA was extracted from swabs of ano-genital or oral ulcers, and PCR product was analyzed by electrophoresis using 2% agarose. The detection limit of PCR was 1 pg *T. pallidum* DNA (~800 organisms). Sensitivities were 94.7% and 80.0% for primary and secondary syphilis, respectively, while specificity was 98.6% for both clinical stages (Palmer et al., 2003). Further, this 260 bp target was used in PCR for detection of *T.pallidum* DNA in latent syphilis by testing whole blood, serum or plasma samples. Ear lobe scraping presented the highest positivity of 51.7% (16/28) followed by plasma, whole blood and serum, with 44.9% (31/69), 39.1% (27/69) and 21.6% (18/69), respectively (Castro et al., 2007).

The PCR based on two unique features of the DNA polymerase I gene (polA) of *T. pallidum* was developed by Liu et al. The first distinctive characteristic is that the region codes for a high cysteine content and has low homology with similar regions of DNA polymerase I gene from known microorganisms. The second unique feature is the presence of four insertions in the gene. PCR tests using primers designed on the basis these regions reacted with various pathogenic *T.pallidum* subspecies but did not react with nonpathogenic treponemal species or other spirochetes. Two sets of primers were used to amplify a fragment of 377 bp (1759-2135) and 395 bp (1539-1933). The detection limit was about 10 to 25 organisms when analyzed on gel, and a single organism when the ABI 310 Prism Genetic

Analyzer was used to detect fluorescence-labeled amplicons. The 112 genital ulcer specimens were tested by polA PCR; sensitivity and specificity was 95.8% and 95.7%, respectively (Liu et al., 2001).

The polA gene of *T.pallidum* was detected in a whole blood from person with syphilis; PCR was positive in 43% (3/7) patients with incubating disease and 62% (8/13) with latent syphilis (Marfin et al., 2001). When used as a screening test for *T. pallidum* DNA detection in lesion samples from patients with clinical diagnosis of syphilis, polA PCR was found positive in 36% (15/42) and 75% (9/12) of samples from patients with primary and secondary syphilis, respectively (Pope et al., 2005).

Martin at al used PCR to amplify the three *T. pallidum* genes: tpp47(Burstain et al., 1991) bmp (Noordhoek et al., 1991) and polA (Liu et al., 2001). PCR was positive in 36%(19/53) specimens, three treponemal gene PCR assays gave concordant results in all specimens collected from syphilis patients, regardless of the specimen types (blood or swab) or the stages of disease (primary or secondary) (Martin et al., 2009). Another study found positivity ratio of 39.1% for ttp47 PCR (260 bp) and 31.1% for polA PCR (378 bp), in blood samples from patients with latent syphilis (Castro et al., 2007).

The real-time PCR had been developed for detection of *T.pallidum* DNA in clinical samples, they targeted polA gene (Heymans et al., 2010; Koek et al., 2006; Leslie et al., 2007) or tpp47 gene (Gayet-Ageron et al., 2009).

The first test was validated using an analytical panel (n = 140) and a clinical panel of genital samples (n = 112) from patients attending a sexually transmitted infections clinic. High sensitivities and specificities of 94-100% were achieved using two real-time PCR platforms, the Rotor-Gene and the iCycler (Koek et al., 2006). Leslie et al developed real-time PCR which analytical sensitivity was estimated to be 1.75 target copies per reaction. Real-time PCR was performed in genital lesion specimens, but not in serum. When compared with serology results, polA gene real-time PCR presented the sensitivity of 80.39% and the specificity of 98.40%(Leslie et al., 2007). Another study found sensitivity of 72.8% and specificity of 95.5% in patients with clinical diagnosis of primary syphilis, the detection of secondary syphilis was low, and the sensitivity was 43.0% (Heymans et al., 2010).

Gayet-Ageron et al evaluated a real-time PCR assay for the detection of tpp47 gene of *T.pallidum* in various biological specimens from patients with primary and secondary syphilis. They found global sensitivity of 65% during primary, 53% during secondary, and null during latent syphilis. Among primary syphilis, real-time PCR positivity was 80% in lesion swabs and 55% in serum, while among secondary syphilis it was 100% in plasma samples (Gayet-Ageron et al., 2009).

In general, PCR presents high sensitivity to detect treponemal DNA in ulcer lesion samples from patients with primary syphilis. *T.pallidum* DNA can be detected in blood samples from patients with latent syphilis, also.

4. Conclusion

The ideal test for syphilis should have both high sensitivity and specifitity, be suitable for monitoring response to treatment, give a negative result after adequate therapy and also give a clear indication of reinfection. Unfortunately, such test does not exist.

PCR methods had been shown high sensitivity for detection of *T.pallidum* DNA in ulcer lesion samples, but lower performance was observed performance in secondary or latent syphilis, probably due to low number of circulating treponemes in these stages.

The new recombinant antigen based automated syphilis assays have the advantage of their high sensitivities in early syphilis and their high throughputs; however as treponemal tests, they cannot distinguish among recent, remote, and previously treated infections. The detection of specific IgM antibodies may be helpful in this issue as it could be detected in active infection including re-infection. Some studies reported a good association between the detection of treponemal specific IgM antibodies and nontreponemal antibodies (VDRL or RPR) in serum samples from patients with untreated syphilis, and also in follow-up of treatment.

POC tests may prove to be effective tools in the control of syphilis and for screening pregnant women to prevent congenital syphilis in primary health care settings, because of its the simplicity and low cost. However, currently available POC tests do not distinguish active and treated syphilis. New POC tests for simultaneous detection of non-treponemal antibodies or for detection of specific IgM antibody developed recently are promising to overcome these limitations.

A great improvement has been achieved for syphilis laboratory diagnosis and it is constantly evolving, but to date, no test is ideal for all stages of syphilis.

5. References

Backhouse, J. L. & Nesteroff, S. I. (2001). Treponema pallidum western blot: Comparison with the FTA-ABS test as a confirmatory test for syphilis. *Diagnostic Microbiology and Infectious Disease* Vol.39, No.1, pp. 9-14, ISSN 0732-8893

Benzaken, A. S., Sabido, M., Galban, E. G., Pedroza, V., Vasquez, F., Araujo, A., Peeling, R. W. & Mayaud, P. (2008). Field evaluation of the performance and testing costs of a rapid point-of-care test for syphilis in a red-light district of Manaus, Brazil. *Sexually Transmitted Infection* Vol.84, No.4, (Aug), pp. 297-302, ISSN 1472-3263

Binnicker, M. J., Jespersen, D. J. & Rollins, L. O. (2011). Treponema-specific tests for serodiagnosis of syphilis: comparative evaluation of seven assays. *Journal of Clinical Microbiology* Vol.49, No.4, (Apr), pp. 1313-1317, ISSN 1098-660X

Bruisten, S. M., Cairo, I., Fennema, H., Pijl, A., Buimer, M., Peerbooms, P. G., Van Dyck, E., Meijer, A., Ossewaarde, J. M. & van Doornum, G. J. (2001). Diagnosing genital ulcer disease in a clinic for sexually transmitted diseases in Amsterdam, The Netherlands. *Journal of Clinical Microbiology* Vol.39, No.2, (Feb), pp. 601-605, ISSN 0095-1137

Burstain, J. M., Grimprel, E., Lukehart, S. A., Norgard, M. V. & Radolf, J. D. (1991). Sensitive detection of Treponema pallidum by using the polymerase chain reaction. *Journal of Clinical Microbiology* Vol.29, No.1, (January 1, 1991), pp. 62-69, ISSN 1098-660X

Castro, A. R., Mody, H. C., Parab, S. Y., Patel, M. T., Kikkert, S. E., Park, M. M. & Ballard, R. C. (2010). An immunofiltration device for the simultaneous detection of non-treponemal and treponemal antibodies in patients with syphilis. *Sexually Transmitted Infections* Vol.86, No.7, (Dec), pp. 532-536, ISSN 1472-3263

Castro, R., Prieto, E., Aguas, M. J., Manata, M. J., Botas, J., Santo, I., Azevedo, J. & Pereira, F. L. H. (2007). Detection of Treponema pallidum sp pallidum DNA in latent syphilis. *International Journal of STD & AIDS* Vol.18, pp. 842-845, ISSN 0956-4624

Centurion-Lara, A., Castro, C., Shaffer, J. M., Van Voorhis, W. C., Marra, C. M. & Lukehart, S. A. (1997). Detection of Treponema pallidum by a sensitive reverse transcriptase PCR. *Journal of Clinical Microbiology*, No.6, (June), pp. 1348-1352, ISSN 1098-660X

Cole, M. J., Perry, K. R. & Parry, J. V. (2007). Comparative evaluation of 15 serological assays for the detection of syphilis infection. *European Journal of Clinical Microbiology and Infectious Disease* Vol.26, No.10, (Oct), pp. 705-713, ISSN 0934-9723

de Lemos, E. A., Belem, Z. R., Santos, A. n. & Ferreira, A. n. W. (2007). Characterization of the Western blotting IgG reactivity patterns in the clinical phases of acquired syphilis. *Diagnostic Microbiology and Infectious Disease* Vol.58, No.2, pp. 177-183, ISSN 1879-0070

Deguchi, M., Hosotsubo, H., Yamashita, N., Ohmine, T. & Asari, S. (1994). Evaluation of gelatin particle agglutination method for detection of Treponema pallidum antibody. *Kansenshogaku Zasshi* Vol.68, No.10, (Oct), pp. 1271-1277, ISSN 0387-5911

Diaz, T., Almeida, M. G., Georg, I., Maia, S. C., De Souza, R. V. & Markowitz, L. E. (2004). Evaluation of the Determine Rapid Syphilis TP assay using sera. *Clinical and Diagnostic Laboratory Immunology* Vol.11, No.1, (Jan), pp. 98-101, ISSN 1071-412X

Ebel, A., Bachelart, L. & Alonso, J. M. (1998). Evaluation of a new competitive immunoassay (BioElisa Syphilis) for screening for Treponema pallidum antibodies at various stages of syphilis. *Journal of Clinical Microbiology* Vol.36, No.2, (Feb), pp. 358-361, ISSN 0095-1137

Ebel, A., Vanneste, L., Cardinaels, M., Sablon, E., Samson, I., De Bosschere, K., Hulstaert, F. & Zrein, M. (2000). Validation of the INNO-LIA syphilis kit as a confirmatory assay for Treponema pallidum antibodies. *Journal of Clinical Microbiology* Vol.38, No.1, (Jan), pp. 215-219, ISSN 0095-1137

Flasarova, M., Smajs, D., Matejkova, P., Woznicova, V., Heroldova-Dvorakova, M. & Votava, M. (2006). Molecular detection and subtyping of Treponema pallidum subsp. pallidum in clinical specimens. *Epidemiologie, Mikrobiologie, Imunologie* Vol.55, No.3, (Aug), pp. 105-111, ISSN 1210-7913

Gayet-Ageron, A., Ninet, B., Toutous-Trellu, L., Lautenschlager, S., Furrer, H., Piguet, V., Schrenzel, J. & Hirschel, B. (2009). Assessment of a real-time PCR test to diagnose syphilis from diverse biological samples. *Sexually Transmitted Infections*, Vol.85, No.4 (Jan), pp.264-269, ISSN 1472-3263

George, R., Pope, V., Fears, M., Morrill, B. & Larsen, S. (1998). An analysis of the value of some antigen-antibody interactions used as diagnostic indicators in a treponemal Western blot (TWB) test for syphilis. *Journal of Clinical and Laboratory Immunology* Vol.50, No.1, pp. 27-44, ISSN 0141-2760

Gianino, M. M., Dal Conte, I., Sciole, K., Galzerano, M., Castelli, L., Zerbi, R., Arnaudo, I., Di Perri, G. & Renga, G. (2007). Performance and costs of a rapid syphilis test in an urban population at high risk for sexually transmitted infections. *Journal of Preventive Medicine and Hygiene* Vol.48, No.4, (Dec), pp. 118-122, ISSN 1121-2233

Gomez, E., Jespersen, D. J., Harring, J. A. & Binnicker, M. J. (2010). Evaluation of the Bio-Rad BioPlex 2200 Syphilis Multiplex Flow Immunoassay for the Detection of IgM- and IgG-Class Antitreponemal Antibodies. *Clinical and Vaccine Immunology* Vol.17, No.6, (Jun), pp. 966-968, ISSN 1556-6811

Grimprel, E., Sanchez, P. J., Wendel, G. D., Burstain, J. M., McCracken, G. H., Jr., Radolf, J. D. & Norgard, M. V. (1991). Use of polymerase chain reaction and rabbit infectivity testing to detect Treponema pallidum in amniotic fluid, fetal and neonatal sera, and cerebrospinal fluid. *Journal of Clinical Microbiology* Vol.29, No.8, (Aug), pp. 1711-1718, ISSN 0095-1137

Gutierrez, J., Vergara, M. J., Soto, M. J., Piedrola, G. & Maroto, M. (2000). Clinical utility of a competitive ELISA to detect antibodies against Treponema pallidum. *Journal of Clinical Laboratory Analysis* Vol.14, No.2, (Feb), pp. 83-86, ISSN 0887-8013

Hagedorn, H. J., Kraminer-Hagedorn, A., De Bosschere, K., Hulstaert, F., Pottel, H. & Zrein, M. (2002). Evaluation of INNO-LIA syphilis assay as a confirmatory test for syphilis. *Journal of Clinical Microbiology* Vol.40, No.3, (Mar), pp. 973-978, ISSN 0095-1137

Halling, V. W., Jones, M. F., Bestrom, J. E., Wold, A. D., Rosenblatt, J. E., Smith, T. F. & Cockerill, F. R., 3rd (1999). Clinical comparison of the Treponema pallidum CAPTIA syphilis-G enzyme immunoassay with the fluorescent treponemal antibody absorption immunoglobulin G assay for syphilis testing. *Journal of Clinical Microbiology* Vol.37, No.10, (Oct), pp. 3233-3234, ISSN 0095-1137

Hay, P. E., Clarke, J. R., Strugnell, R. A., Taylor-Robinson, D. & Goldmeier, D. (1990a). Use of the polymerase chain reaction to detect DNA sequences specific to pathogenic treponemes in cerebrospinal fluid. *FEMS Microbiology Letters.* Vol.56, No.3, (Mar), pp. 233-238, ISSN 0378-1097

Hay, P. E., Clarke, J. R., Taylor-Robinson, D. & Goldmeier, D. (1990b). Detection of treponemal DNA in the CSF of patients with syphilis and HIV infection using the polymerase chain reaction. *Genitourinary Medicine* Vol.66, No.6, (Dec), pp. 428-432, ISSN 0266-4348

Herring, A. J., Ballard, R. C., Pope, V., Adegbola, R. A., Changalucha, J., Fitzgerald, D. W., Hook, E. W., Kubanova, A., Mananwatte, S., Pape, J. W., Sturm, A. W., West, B., Yin, Y. P. & Peeling, R. W. (2006). A multi-centre evaluation of nine rapid, point-of-care syphilis tests using archived sera. *Sexually Transmitted Infections* Vol.82, No.suppl 5, (Dec), pp. 7-12, ISSN 1472-3263

Heymans, R., van der Helm, J. J., de Vries, H. J. C., Fennema, H. S. A., Coutinho, R. A. & Bruisten, S. M. (2010). Clinical Value of Treponema pallidum Real-Time PCR for Diagnosis of Syphilis. *Journal of Clinical Microbiology* Vol.48, No.2, (Feb), pp. 497-502, ISSN 0095-1137

Hook, E. W. & Marra, C. M. (1992). Acquired Syphilis in Adults. *New England Journal of Medicine* Vol.326, No.16, (Apr), pp. 1060-1069, ISSN 0028-4793

Jurado, R. L., Campbell, J. & Martin, P. D. (1993). Prozone Phenomenon in Secondary Syphilis: Has Its Time Arrived? *Archives of Internal Medicine* Vol.153, No.21, (Nov), pp. 2496-2498, ISSN 0003-9926

Knight, C. S., Crum, M. A. & Hardy, R. W. (2007). Evaluation of the LIAISON chemiluminescence immunoassay for diagnosis of syphilis. *Clinical and Vaccine Immunology* Vol.14, No.6, (Jun), pp. 710-713, ISSN 1556-679X

Koek, A. G., Bruisten, S. M., Dierdorp, M., van Dam, A. P. & Templeton, K. (2006). Specific and sensitive diagnosis of syphilis using a real-time PCR for Treponema pallidum.

Clinical Microbiology and Infection Vol.12, No.12, (Dec), pp. 1233-1236, ISSN 1469-0691

Kouznetsov, A. V. & Prinz, J. C. (2002). Molecular diagnosis of syphilis: the Schaudinn-Hoffmann lymph-node biopsy. *The Lancet* Vol.360, No.9330, (Aug), pp. 388-389, ISSN 0140-6736

Kouznetsov, A. V., Weisenseel, P., Trommler, P., Multhaup, S. & Prinz, J. C. (2005). Detection of the 47-kilodalton membrane immunogen gene of Treponema pallidum in various tissue sources of patients with syphilis. *Diagnostic Microbiology and Infectious Disease* Vol.51, No.2, (Feb), pp. 143-145, ISSN 0732-8893

Lam, T. K., Lau, H. Y., Lee, Y. P., Fung, S. M., Leung, W. L. & Kam, K. M. (2010). Comparative evaluation of the INNO-LIA syphilis score and the MarDx Treponema pallidum immunoglobulin G Marblot test assays for the serological diagnosis of syphilis. *International Journal of STD & AIDS* Vol.21, No.2, (Feb), pp. 110-113, ISSN 0956-4624

Larsen S.A., Hunter E.F. & Kraus S.J., (1990). *A Manual of tests for syphilis*, (8th Ed.) Washington, DC : American Public Health Association, pp.191 ISBN 0875531741

Larsen, S. A., Steiner, B. M. & Rudolph, A. H. (1995). Laboratory diagnosis and interpretation of tests for syphilis. *Clinical Microbiology Reviews.* Vol.8, No.1, (Jan), pp. 1-21, ISSN 0893-8512

Lefevre, J. C., Bertrand, M. A. & Bauriaud, R. (1990). Evaluation of the Captia enzyme immunoassays for detection of immunoglobulins G and M to Treponema pallidum in syphilis. *Journal of Clinical Microbiology* Vol.28, No.8, (Aug), pp. 1704-1707, ISSN 0095-1137

Leslie, D. E., Azzato, F., Karapanagiotidis, T., Leydon, J. & Fyfe, J. (2007). Development of a Real-Time PCR Assay To Detect Treponema pallidum in Clinical Specimens and Assessment of the Assay's Performance by Comparison with Serological Testing. *Journal of Clinical Microbiology* Vol.45, No.1, (Jan), pp. 93-96, ISSN 1098-660X

Li, J., Zheng, H. Y., Wang, L. N., Liu, Y. X., Wang, X. F. & Liu, X. R. (2009). Clinical evaluation of four recombinant Treponema pallidum antigen-based rapid diagnostic tests for syphilis. *Journal of the European Academy of Dermatology and Venereology* Vol.23, No.6, (Jun), pp. 648-650, ISSN 1468-3083

Lin, L.-R., Tong, M.-L., Fu, Z.-G., Dan, B., Zheng, W.-H., Zhang, C.-G., Yang, T.-C. & Zhang, Z.-Y. (2011). Evaluation of a colloidal gold immunochromatography assay in the detection of Treponema pallidum specific IgM antibody in syphilis serofast reaction patients: a serologic marker for the relapse and infection of syphilis. *Diagnostic Microbiology and Infectious Disease* Vol.70, No.1, (May) pp. 10-16, ISSN 1879-0070

Liu, H., Rodes, B., Chen, C. Y. & Steiner, B. (2001). New Tests for Syphilis: Rational Design of a PCR Method for Detection of Treponema pallidum in Clinical Specimens Using Unique Regions of the DNA Polymerase I Gene. *Journal of Clinical Microbiology* Vol.39, No.5, (May), pp. 1941-1946, ISSN 1098-660X

Mabey, D., Peeling, R. W., Ballard, R., Benzaken, A. S., GalbÃ¡n, E., Changalucha, J., Everett, D., Balira, R., Fitzgerald, D., Joseph, P., Nerette, S., Li, J. & Zheng, H. (2006a). Prospective, multi-centre clinic-based evaluation of four rapid diagnostic tests for syphilis. *Sexually Transmitted Infections* Vol.82, No.suppl 5, (Dec), pp. v13-v16, ISSN 1368-4973

Maidment, C., Woods, A. & Chan, R. (1998). An evaluation of the Behring Diagnostics Enzygnost Syphilis enzyme immunoassay. *Pathology* Vol.30, No.2, (May), pp. 177-178, ISSN 0031-3025

Manavi, K. & McMillan, A. (2007). The outcome of treatment of early latent syphilis and syphilis with undetermined duration in HIV-infected and HIV-uninfected patients. *International Journal of Std & Aids* Vol.18, No.12, (Dec), pp. 814-818, ISSN 0956-4624

Marangoni, A., Sambri, V., Accardo, S., Cavrini, F., D'Antuono, A., Moroni, A., Storni, E. & Cevenini, R. (2005). Evaluation of LIAISON Treponema Screen, a Novel Recombinant Antigen-Based Chemiluminescence Immunoassay for Laboratory Diagnosis of Syphilis. *Clinical and Diagnostic Laboratory Immunology.* Vol.12, No.10, (Oct), pp. 1231-1234, ISSN 1098-6588

Marangoni A., Moroni A., Accardo, S. & Cevenini, R. (2009). Laboratory diagnosis of syphilis with automated immunoassays. *Journal of Clinical Laboratory Analysis* Vol.23, No.1, (Jan), pp. 1-6, ISSN 1098-2825

Marfin, A. A., Liu, H., Sutton, M. Y., Steiner, B., Pillay, A. & Markowitz, L. E. (2001). Amplification of the DNA polymerase I gene of Treponema pallidum from whole blood of persons with syphilis. *Diagnostic Microbiology and Infectious Disease* Vol.40, No.4, (Aug) pp. 163-166, ISSN 0732-8893

Martin, I. E., Tsang, R. S. W., Sutherland, K., Tilley, P., Read, R., Anderson, B., Roy, C. & Singh, A. E. (2009). Molecular Characterization of Syphilis in Patients in Canada: Azithromycin Resistance and Detection of Treponema pallidum DNA in Whole-Blood Samples versus Ulcerative Swabs. *Journal of Clinical Microbiology* Vol.47, No.6, (Jun), pp. 1668-1673, ISSN 1098-660X

McMillan, A. & Young, H. (2008). Reactivity in the Venereal Diseases Research Laboratory test and the Mercia(R) IgM enzyme immunoassay after treatment of early syphilis. *International Journal of Std & Aids* Vol.19, No.10, (Oct), pp. 689-693, ISSN 0956-4624

Mishra, S., Naik, B., Venugopal, B., Kudur, P., Washington, R., Becker, M., Kenneth, J., Jayanna, K., Ramesh, B. M., Isac, S., Boily, M. C., Blanchard, J. F. & Moses, S. (2010). Syphilis screening among female sex workers in Bangalore, India: comparison of point-of-care testing and traditional serological approaches. *Sexually Transmitted Infections* Vol.86, No.3, (Jun), pp. 193-198, ISSN 1472-3263

Montoya, P. J., Lukehart, S. A., Brentlinger, P. E., Blanco, A. J., Floriano, F., Sairosse, J. & Gloyd, S. (2006). Comparison of the diagnostic accuracy of a rapid immunochromatographic test and the rapid plasma reagin test for antenatal syphilis screening in Mozambique. *Bulletin of World Health Organization* Vol.84, No.2, (Feb), pp. 97-104, ISSN 0042-9686

Noordhoek, G. T., Wolters, E. C., de Jonge, M. E. & van Embden, J. D. (1991). Detection by polymerase chain reaction of Treponema pallidum DNA in cerebrospinal fluid from neurosyphilis patients before and after antibiotic treatment. *Journal of Clinical Microbiology.* Vol.29, No.9, (Sep), pp. 1976-1984, ISSN 0095-1137

Orle, K. A., Gates, C. A., Martin, D. H., Body, B. A. & Weiss, J. B. (1996). Simultaneous PCR detection of Haemophilus ducreyi, Treponema pallidum, and herpes simplex virus types 1 and 2 from genital ulcers. *Journal of Clinical Microbiology.* Vol.34, No.1, (Jan), pp. 49-54, ISSN 1098-660X

Oshiro, M., Taira, R., Kyan, T. & Yamane, N. (1999). Laboratory-based evaluation of DainaScreen TPAb to detect specific antibodies against Treponema pallidum. *Rinsho Biseibutshu Jinsoku Shindan Kenkyukai Shi* Vol.10, No.1, pp. 27-32, ISSN 0915-1753

Palmer, H. M., Higgins, S. P., Herring, A. J. & Kingston, M. A. (2003). Use of PCR in the diagnosis of early syphilis in the United Kingdom. *Sexually Transmitted Infectious* Vol.79, No.6, (Dec), pp. 479-483, ISSN 1368-4973

Pope, V., Fears, M. B., Morrill, W. E., Castro, A. & Kikkert, S. E. (2000). Comparison of the Serodia Treponema pallidum particle agglutination, Captia Syphilis-G, and SpiroTek Reagin II tests with standard test techniques for diagnosis of syphilis. *Journal of Clinical Microbiology*Vol.38, No.7, (Jul), pp. 2543-2545, ISSN 0095-1137

Pope, V., Fox, K., Liu, H., Marfin, A. A., Leone, P., Sena, A. C., Chapin, J., Fears, M. B. & Markowitz, L. (2005). Molecular Subtyping of Treponema pallidum from North and South Carolina. *Journal of Clinical Microbiology* Vol.43, No.8, (Aug), pp. 3743-3746, ISSN 1098-660X

Rathlev, T. (1967). Haemagglutination test utilizing pathogenic Treponema pallidum for the sero-diagnosis of syphilis. *The British Journal of Venereal Diseases*Vol.43, No.3, (Sep), pp. 181-185, ISSN 0007-134X

Rotty, J., Anderson, D., Garcia, M., Diaz, J., Van de Waarsenburg, S., Howard, T., Dennison, A., Lewin, S. R., Elliott, J. H. & Hoy, J. (2010). Preliminary assessment of Treponema pallidum-specific IgM antibody detection and a new rapid point-of-care assay for the diagnosis of syphilis in human immunodeficiency virus-1-infected patients. *International Journal of Std & Aids* Vol.21, No.11, (Nov), pp. 758-764, ISSN 1758-1052

Rudolph, A. H. (1976). The microhemagglutination assay for Treponema pallidum antibodies (MHA-TP), a new treponemal test for syphilis: where does it fit? *Journal of the American Venereal Disease Association* Vol.3, No.1, (Sep), pp. 3-8, ISSN 0095-148X

Sanchez, P. J., Wendel, G. D., Jr., Grimprel, E., Goldberg, M., Hall, M., Arencibia-Mireles, O., Radolf, J. D. & Norgard, M. V. (1993). Evaluation of molecular methodologies and rabbit infectivity testing for the diagnosis of congenital syphilis and neonatal central nervous system invasion by Treponema pallidum. *The Journal of Infectious Diseases* Vol.167, No.1, (Jan), pp. 148-157, ISSN 0022-1899

Sato, N. S., de Melo, C. S., Zerbini, L. C., Silveira, E. P., Fagundes, L. J. & Ueda, M. (2003). Assessment of the rapid test based on an immunochromatography technique for detecting anti-Treponema pallidum antibodies. *Revista do Instituto de Medicina Tropical de Sao Paulo* Vol.45, No.6, (Nov-Dec), pp. 319-322, ISSN 0036-4665 Sato, N. S., Suzuki, T., Ueda, T., Watanabe, K., Hirata, R. D. & Hirata, M. H. (2004). Recombinant antigen-based immuno-slot blot method for serodiagnosis of syphilis. *Brazilian Journal Medical Biology Research* Vol.37, No.7, (Jul), pp. 949-955, ISSN 0100-879X

Schmidt, B. L., Edjlalipour, M. & Luger, A. (2000). Comparative evaluation of nine different enzyme-linked immunosorbent assays for determination of antibodies against

Treponema pallidum in patients with primary syphilis. *Journal of Clinical Microbiology*Vol.38, No.3, (Mar), pp. 1279-1282, ISSN 0095-1137

Siedner, M., Zapitz, V., Ishida, M., De La Roca, R. & Klausner, J. D. (2004). Performance of rapid syphilis tests in venous and fingerstick whole blood specimens. *Sexually Transmitted Diseases* Vol.31, No.9, (Sep), pp. 557-560, ISSN 0148-5717

Silletti, R. P. (1995). Comparison of CAPTIA syphilis G enzyme immunoassay with rapid plasma reagin test for detection of syphilis. *Journal of Clinical Microbiology* Vol.33, No.7, (Jul), pp. 1829-1831, ISSN 0095-1137

Tinajeros, F., Grossman, D., Richmond, K., Steele, M., Garcia, S. G., Zegarra, L. & Revollo, R. (2006). Diagnostic accuracy of a point-of-care syphilis test when used among pregnant women in Bolivia. *Sexually Transmitted Infections* Vol.82 Suppl 5, (Dec), pp. v17-21, ISSN 1368-4973

Tomizawa, T. (1966). Hemagglutination tests for diagnosis of syphilis. A preliminary report. *Japanese Journal of Medical Science & Biology*. Vol.19, No.6, (Dec), pp. 305-308, ISSN 0021-5112

Tsang, R. S., Martin, I. E., Lau, A. & Sawatzky, P. (2007). Serological diagnosis of syphilis: comparison of the Trep-Chek IgG enzyme immunoassay with other screening and confirmatory tests. *FEMS Immunology and Medical Microbiology* Vol.51, No.1, (Oct), pp. 118-124, 0928-8244

Veldkamp, J. & Visser, A. M. (1975). Application of the enzyme-linked immunosorbent assay (ELISA) in the serodiagnosis of syphilis. *The British Journal of Venereal Diseases* Vol.51, No.4, (Aug), pp. 227-231, ISSN 0007-134X

Viriyataveekul, R., Laodee, N., Potprasat, S. & Piyophirapong, S. (2006). Comparative evaluation of three different treponemal enzyme immunoassays for syphilis. *Journal of the Medical Association of Thailand* Vol.89, No.6, (Jun), pp. 773-779, ISSN 0125-2208

Welch, R. J. & Litwin, C. M. (2010). Evaluation of two immunoblot assays and a Western blot assay for the detection of antisyphilis immunoglobulin g antibodies. *Clinical and Vaccine Immunology* : Vol.17, No.1, (Jan), pp. 183-184, ISSN 1556-679X

Wellinghausen, N. & Dietenberger, H. (2011). Evaluation of two automated chemiluminescence immunoassays, the LIAISON Treponema Screen and the ARCHITECT Syphilis TP, and the Treponema pallidum particle agglutination test for laboratory diagnosis of syphilis. *Clinical Chemistry and Laboratory Medicine* Vol.49, No.8, (Aug), pp. 1375-1377, ISSN 1434-6621

Woznicova, V. & Valisova, Z. (2007). Performance of CAPTIA SelectSyph-G enzyme-linked immunosorbent assay in syphilis testing of a high-risk population: analysis of discordant results. *Journal of Clinical Microbiology* Vol.45, No.6, (Jun), pp. 1794-1797, ISSN 0095-1137

Yoshioka, N., Deguchi, M., Kagita, M., Kita, M., Watanabe, M., Asari, S. & Iwatani, Y. (2007). Evaluation of a chemiluminescent microparticle immunoassay for determination of Treponema pallidum antibodies. *Clinical Laboratory* Vol.53, No.9-12, (Dec), pp. 597-603, ISSN 1433-6510

Young, H., Moyes, A., McMillan, A. & Robertson, D. H. (1989). Screening for treponemal infection by a new enzyme immunoassay. *Genitourinary Medicine* Vol.65, No.2, (Apr), pp. 72-78, ISSN 0266-4348

Young, H., Moyes, A., Seagar, L. & McMillan, A. (1998). Novel recombinant-antigen enzyme immunoassay for serological diagnosis of syphilis. *Journal of Clinical Microbiology* Vol.36, No.4, (Apr), pp. 913-917, ISSN 0095-1137

Young, H., Pryde, J., Duncan, L. & Dave, J. (2009). The Architect Syphilis assay for antibodies to Treponema pallidum: an automated screening assay with high sensitivity in primary syphilis. *Sexually Transmitted Infections* Vol.85, No.1, (Feb), pp. 19-23, ISSN 1368-4973

Young, H., Walker, P. J., Merry, D. & Mifsud, A. (1994). A preliminary evaluation of a prototype western blot confirmatory test kit for syphilis. *International Journal of STD & AIDS* Vol.5, No.6, (Nov-Dec), pp. 409-414, ISSN 0956-4624

7

Serologic Response to Treatment in Syphilis

Neuza Satomi Sato
Center of Immunology, Institute Adolfo Lutz
São Paulo, SP
Brazil

1. Introduction

Serologic monitoring is the way to determine adequate treatment response, which is typically defined as a fourfold decline in Rapid Plasma Reagin (RPR) or Veneral Disease Research Laboratory (VDRL) titer within 6 months of treatment for patients with primary or secondary syphilis and within 12 months of treatment for patients with early latent syphilis. Studies documented close to 100% rate seroreversion 1 -2 years after penicillin treatment, depending on the stage of syphilis and duration of symptoms.

HIV co-infection has several effects on the presentation, diagnosis, disease progression, and therapy of syphilis. Unusual syphilis serologic titers have been reported in HIV-infected patients, with either unexpected high or low titer, as well as delayed serologic response at the time of diagnosis. There are several studies concerned to syphilis serological treatment response comparing HIV-infected and HIV-negative patients. Some studies reported a slower serological response in HIV infected patients. A recent study showed that the use of high active antiretroviral therapy (HAART) and the routine use of macrolides for the prevention of opportunistic infections may reduce syphilis serologic failure rates among HIV-infected patients who have syphilis.

Penicillin G, administered parenterally, is the preferred drug for treating all stages of syphilis (French et al., 2009; Workowski & Berman, 2010). Treatment failure can occur with any regimen. Assessing response to treatment frequently is difficult, and definitive criteria for cure or failure have not been established.

According to the CDC guidelines recommendations, clinical and serologic evaluation should be performed 6 months and 12 months after treatment of patients with primary or secondary syphilis; more frequent evaluation might be prudent if follow-up is uncertain.

Patients who have signs or symptoms that persists or recurs or who have sustained fourfold increase in nontreponemal test titer probably failed treatment or were reinfected. The latent syphilis is not transmitted sexually; the objective of treating patients with this stage of disease is to prevent complication. Quantitative nontreponemal serologic tests should be repeated at 6, 12, and 24 months for follow- up. Limited information is available concerning clinical and serological follow-up of patients who have tertiary syphilis. HIV-infected persons should be evaluated clinically and serologically for treatment failure at 3, 6, 9, 12, and 24 months after therapy (Workowski & Berman, 2010).

Usually, treatment failure cannot be distinguished from reinfection with *T. pallidum*; in these cases a CSF analysis is recommended.

2. Serorevertion of the serological tests for syphilis

Patients treated for syphilis are monitored by quantitative nontreponemal tests (VDRL or RPR). The rate of decrease of serologic titers is influenced by many factors, including the history of previous syphilis, the stage of infection, the baseline serologic titers, the immune status, and the administered treatment (Augenbraun et al., 1998; Brown et al., 1999; Fiumara, 1977a, 1977b, 1978; Ghanem et al., 2007; Romanowski et al., 1987; Talwar et al., 1992).

2.1 Nontreponemal antibodies

Nontreponemal test antibody titers may correlate with disease activity, and results should be reported quantitatively. Nontreponemal test titers usually declines after treatment and might become nonreactive with time, however, in some persons, these antibodies can persist for a long period of time, a response referred to as the serofast reaction (Workowski & Berman, 2010).

In a study of 586 patients with early syphilis treated with benzathine penicillin, 2.4 mU, the VDRL was nonreactive in 97% of patients with primary syphilis and 77% with secondary syphilis, within 2 years (Schroeter et al., 1972).

Fiumara carried a series of studies of serologic response to treatment in patients at different stage of syphilis disease. A study of 588 patients with primary syphilis found that all patients were seronegative after 1 year, and all 623 with secondary syphilis had seroreverted their nontreponemal tests within within 2 years. A study which included 275 early latent syphilis patients of less than one year duration, demonstrated that all but 2 of the patients became seronegative within 4 years. In another study of 123 patients with late latent syphilis, 44% became seronegative within five years, and 56% had persistently positive nontreponemal tests (Fiumara, 1979). Most of the patients in these studies were treated with higher dose of penicillin than currently recommended (Workowski & Berman, 2010), and the rest of the patients were treated with tetracycline.

A study of serologic response in a cohort of 818 patients treated for primary or secondary syphilis found that VDRL titer declined approximately fourfold at 3 months and eightfold at 6 months. The serological response of patients treated with erythromycin was inferior to that achieved by penicillin or tetracycline (Brown et al., 1999).

Anderson et al. reported that in most patients the VDRL test showed a consistent fall in titer after treatment, however a small proportion continued to give positive results with no evidence of reinfection or treatment fail (Anderson et al., 1989). The study analyzed data from 946 patients with primary and 854 patients with secondary syphilis, and follow-up serology by VDRL was carried at 6 and 18 months. Of the patients with primary syphilis, seroreversion were found in 70% and 85%, respectively at 6 and 18 months. Patients with secondary syphilis, 45% became seronegative within 6 months and 68% at 18 months. Treatment most often used was intramuscular procaine penicillin (> 85%), benzathine penicillin was used in only approximately 3% of patients, and non-penicillin drugs included erythromycin or tetracycline. No significant differences were found comparing titers in patients treated with penicillin or non-penicillin (Anderson et al., 1989).

The serologic response was evaluated in a historical cohort study of patients treated for syphilis from 1981 to 1987 in Alberta, Canada. A total of 882 patients included in the analyses were treated with the currently recommended benzathine penicillin regimens. After 3 years, 72% and 56% of patients with initial primary and secondary syphilis had seroreversal of RPR tests. A fourfold decrease and a sixfold decrease were seen in patients with primary and secondary syphilis by 6 and 12 months, respectively, while a fourfold decline was seen in patients with early latent syphilis by 12 months. Serologic response was not affected by gender, age, race, or sexual orientation. Patients with their first infection were more likely to experience RPR seroreversion than those with repeat infections (Singh & Romanowski, 1999).

In a retrospective study of 1,532 patients with early syphilis, the majority of seropositive cases had nonreactive VDRL by 6 months after treatment. Seroreversion was observed in 84% of patients with primary syphilis, 72% of patients with secondary syphilis, and 81% of patients with early latent syphilis by 6 months. The percentages were 93, 92, and 88%, respectively at the end of the 30 months study period. Approximately 86% of patients were treated with benzathine penicillin, 2.4 mU. Others were treated with higher doses of benzathine penicillin, 4.8 mU, and procaine penicillin, which appeared to accelerate the speed of seroconversion (Talwar et al., 1992).

2.2 Anti-treponemal antibodies

Treponemal test antibody titers should not be used to assess treatment response. Most patients who have reactive treponemal tests will have reactive tests for the reminder of their lives, regardless of treatment or disease activity.

However, the disappearance of reactivity in the treponemal tests after treatment of immunocompetent patients and over time has been reported. Schoeter et al. reported that 14% of patients with early syphilis lost their reactivity in the FTA-abs test within 2 years after treatment (Schroeter et al., 1972). Another study demonstrated that in patients with first episode syphilis, 24% of had a non-reactive FTA-abs and 13% had a nonreactive MHA-Tp in 3 years (Romanowski et al., 1991). A prospective, cohort treatment study of 261 patients with early syphilis that had 1 year serologic follow-up with FTA-abs or MHA-TP found seroreversion in 9% and 5% of cases, respectively. No association between HIV-seropositivity and treponemal specific test seroreversion was demonstrated (Augenbraun et al., 1998). Castro et al. performed a study of serologic follow-up of small number of patients with early syphilis. Of the 54 patients evaluated 6 months after therapy, 70% had at least twofold titer decrease when using the specific passive agglutination test (TP.PA); only 22 patients returned for 12 months evaluation, and 19 (86%) had decreased antibody titer. Seroreversion for anti-treponemal antibodies were not found in this study (Castro et al., 2001).

Other studies were performed by Western Blot technique, which provides analyses of reactivity against each specific antigenic fraction. Kim et al. observed a significant loss of anti-Tp47 after treatment of primary syphilis, with complete seroreversion in 11 months (Kim et al., 1989). George group studied 124 persons with clinically diagnosed syphilis by using densitometric quantization and spreadsheet normalization to refine the parameters defining treponemal WB for syphilis. The reactivity against Tp47 was 100% before treatment, while 28% had lost anti-Tp47 over 12 months after treatment (Fraser et al., 1998). More studies are necessary to state if a specific treponemal protein can be used as a potential marker for monitoring treatment.

2.3 Specific IgM

For long time, the utility of IgM in the diagnosis of syphilis has been discussed. Although there have been multiple studies addressing the use of IgM, the results have conflicted somewhat. In the past, a study for quantitative evaluation of the FTA-abs-IgM and VDRL in treated and untreated syphilis revealed sera remained reactive with increased titers for more than one year after treatment in 19.5% patients with primary and 15% patients with secondary syphilis. In follow-up of nine patients with secondary syphilis, FTA-abs-IgM and VDRL titers showed only partial agreement during the course of observation. The FTA-abs-IgM titer usually reverted to non-reactivity later than de VDRL dilutions, indicating that VDRL was better for monitoring treatment (Luger et al., 1977).

Actually, the results of specific IgM tests, either by Western Blot or ELISA for capture of IgM, are essential in the diagnosis of congenital syphilis as well as in the recognition of re-infection; they indicate the need for treatment and are useful in the assessment of the effectiveness of therapy (Schmidt et al., 1994).

McMillan & Young analyzed reactivity in VDRL test and Mercia IgM-Elisa (IgM-EIA) after treatment of 229 patients with early syphilis. The seroreversion observed for IgM-EIA and VDRL were respectively 62% and 41%, at 3 months follow-up, and 1 year after treatment the IgM-EIA were negative in 92% patients while VDRL were negative in 70% cases. A fourfold or greater decrease in VDRL titer occurred in 99% of patient at 3 and 12 months. It was concluded that the Mercia IgM EIA is as sensitive as VDRL in monitoring treatment of primary syphilis, but not as sensitive as the finding of a fourfold or eightfold decrease in VDRL titer in patients treated for secondary or early latent infection (McMillan & Young, 2008).

A study to evaluate *Treponema pallidum*-specific IgM as marker of infectious syphilis in human immunodeficiency virus (HIV)-infected patients was performed with 20 samples from HIV-infected patients with untreated syphilis and follow-up at 3, 6 or 12 months after treatment. The IgM detection detection by Mercia-EIA appears to be a reliable marker for untreated syphilis in HIV-infected patients with primary or secondary syphilis. After treatment, IgM was no longer detected after three months in the majority of patients (87%) and was either negative or equivocal in all patients after six and 12 months (Rotty et al., 2010). It has also been suggested that detection of syphilis specific IgM may correlate with active disease and assist in differentiating active from past and successfully treated syphilis.

3. Syphilis in HIV-infected patients

For most HIV-infected persons, serologic tests are accurate and reliable for the diagnosis of syphilis and for following a patient's response to treatment. However, atypical syphilis serologic tests results can occur in HIV-infected persons. Most reports have involved serologic titers that were higher than expected, but false-negative and delayed appearance of seroreactivity or fluctuating titers also have been reported (Palmer et al., 2003).

When serologic test do not correspond with clinical findings suggestive of early syphilis, use of others tests should be considered, such as biopsy, darkfield microscopy or polymerase chain reaction.

Besides studies of syphilis serologic response rate, several authors have evaluated the time to serologic response according to HIV status, with conflicting results. Some studies found a slower serologic response in HIV infected patients, but other did not. Also, a higher risk of serological failure was associated with HIV infection (Ghanem et al., 2007; Gonzalez-Lopez et al., 2009; Kofoed et al., 2006; Malone et al., 1995; Telzak et al., 1991; Walter et al., 2006; Yinnon et al., 1996).

Neurosyphilis should be considered in the differential diagnosis of neurological disease in HIV-infected person. For patients whose nontreponemal test titers do not decrease fourfold within 6-12 months therapy, CSF examination and retreatment also should be strongly considered (Workowski & Berman, 2010).

3.1 Pre-HAART

According to CDC guidelines, HIV infected person should be evaluated clinically and serologically for treatment failure at 3, 6, 9, 12 and 24 months. If after therapy, nontreponemal titers do not decline fourfold during 12-24 months or titers rise fourfold, at any time, it might be indicative of treatment failure. A higher risk of serological failure was associated with HIV infection.

Telzak et al. performed a retrospective review of response to standard therapy in HIV-infected patients with primary or secondary syphilis. They reported that in patients with primary syphilis, HIV infected patients were less likely to have a fourfold or greater RPR decrease or seroreversion within 6 months of treatment compared with HIV negative patients ($P = 0.03$). Patients with secondary syphilis had similar serological response after treatment, regardless of HIV status (Telzak et al., 1991).

Malone et al reported a relapse or failure rate of 18% in 56 HIV positive patients with follow-up for a mean of 28 months. Relapse occurred more than 12 months after initial therapy in 6 of 10 patients (60%) who experienced relapse; 5 patients experienced multiple relapses. Treatment failure was not related with CD4 count or to a specific antimicrobial regimen. However, the results suggest that patients with clinical evidence of secondary syphilis or with reactive cerebrospinal fluid VDRL test titers were at highest risk of subsequent relapse or treatment failure when monitored for an average of 2 years (Malone et al., 1995).

Rolfs et al. performed a study of randomized trial of enhanced therapy for early syphilis in 541 patients including 101 patients who had HIV infection. Patients were treated with 2.4 mU benzathine penicillin G with or without enhanced therapy consisting of 2 g of amoxicillin and 500 mg of probenecid 3 times daily for 10 days. After 1 year follow-up, 14% of patients were serologically defined as treatment failures; the serologic failure rate was higher in HIV infected patients. Enhanced treatment with amoxicillin and probenecid did not improve the outcomes, and the authors concluded that CDC recommendations for treating early syphilis are adequate for most patients, whether or not they have HIV infection (Augenbraun et al., 1998).

Ghanem and collaborators performed a comparative study of serological response to syphilis treatment in 129 HIV positive and 168 HIV negative patients attending sexually transmitted diseases clinics between 1992 and 2000. Serologic failure was defined as lack of a fourfold drop in RPR titer by 400 days after treatment or a fourfold increase titer between 30 and 400 days. They found 22 serologic failure (17%) in HIV positive groups and 5 in HIV negative group ($p < 0.001$). The median times to successful serological responses were 278 and 126 days, respectively for HIV positive and HIV negative groups ($p < 0.001$). The difference in serologic failure rates was significant in the subgroup of early syphilis, while the difference in median times to successful serologic response was also significant in the subgroup of late latent syphilis. A higher risk of serologic failure was associated with HIV infection (Ghanem et al., 2007).

A study of 41 cases of syphilis diagnosed in HIV-1 infected patients revealed treatment failure in 10% (4 patients) in 7 months follow-up. Also, syphilis was associated with decrease in CD4 cell count and an increase in HIV-RNA levels, and both improved after syphilis treatment (Kofoed et al., 2006). The evaluation of 64 HIV seropositive patients and matched controls retrieved a slower serologic response in HIV infected patients. The HIV-positive patients with initial RPR less than 1:32 experienced a significantly slower decrease in RPR at 12 months than did the controls ($P < .001$) (Yinnon et al., 1996).

Another study by Agmon-Levin et al. analyzed response to recommended treatments of 81 patients which completed 12 months follow-up. Treatment success was documented in 26%, a high rate of serofast (41%) and treatment failure (33%) were found. The immune response correlated with immune status of the patients, the mean CD4 counts were higher and HIV viral load were lower in patients with successful treatments (Agmon-Levin et al., 2010). The increased prevalence of serofast reaction has been reported in co-infected patients previously. This might be attributed to HIV associated hyperglobulinaemia or a longer period of time (2-5 years) required for VDRL levels to decline in HIV infected patients, especially those with prolonged infection or low VDRL levels, lower than 1:8 (Manavi & McMillan, 2007).

González-López et al. performed a longitudinal, retrospective study in a cohort of HIV positive and HIV negative patients with syphilis. Serologic failure was observed in 29.6% (37/125) of HIV positive patients and 11.2% (7/62) HIV negative patients (odds ratio, 3.3; $p < 0.05$). A slower serologic response to treatment was demonstrated in men HIV infected patients with late stage syphilis. HIV negative patients responded more frequently to treatment, but after 2 years follow-up, both groups shared similar response rates (Gonzalez-Lopez et al., 2009). Another study found that HIV infected patients had greater rate of incident syphilis compared with HIV uninfected. Also, HIV infected patients had a greater likelihood to decline in RPR test titer and serologic failure (Horberg et al., 2010).

Others reported no association between serologic failure for syphilis treatment and patient's HIV status. Manavi et al. performed a study to compare outcome of syphilis treatment in HIV infected and uninfected patients. Patients with diagnosis of syphilis who had 24 months follow-up syphilis serology included 161 HIV negative and 129 HIV positive patients. The lack fourfold decrease of VDRL test titer within 12 months in absence of history of re-infection was considered as treatment failure. After 12 months, 63% of HIV negative and 70% of HIV positive patients were treated ($p = 0.04$). HIV serologic status were not associated with success of treatment, and treatment failure in a proportion of HIV positive patients was due to slower decline in VDRL titer rather than lack of response to treatment (Manavi & McMillan, 2007).

Seroreversion of reactive antibodies in patients previously treated for syphilis have been reported in patients with AIDS (Haas et al., 1990; Johnson et al., 1991). Haas analyzed sera from 90 HIV positive and 19 HIV negative men observed for a mean follow-up of 4 years. None of the HIV seronegative individuals lost reactivity to a treponemal test, whereas 7% of the seropositive asymptomatic individuals and 38% of those with symptomatic HIV infection had loss of reactivity. Symptomatic HIV infection was associated with loss of reactivity, as a CD4 count less than 200 cells/uL, a CD4/CD8 ratio less than 0.6, a single prior episode of syphilis, and a low VDRL titer at the time of the last documented episode of syphilis (Haas et al., 1990). Johnson found that 10% (3/29) patients with AIDS had loss of reactivity for both the hemagglutination (TPHA) and FTA-abs over a period of 3 years;

whereas no seroreversion was observed in the 29 controls (Johnson et al., 1991). Janier et al evaluated the long-term outcome of syphilis treponemal tests in a cohort of HIV positive male homosexuals with a history of treated syphilis (69 patients) as compared with HIV negative controls (49 patients). The decrease in VDRL titers was not different between 2 groups (p = 0.053). Time to seroreversion was shorter in HIV positive patients for TPHA (p = 0.009) and FTA-abs test (p = 0.001). The seroreversion of the FTA-abs test was related to a low baseline CD4 cell count (p = 0. 003), while the seroreversion of TPHA and VDRL were not related. After adjustment for the CD4 cell count, only TPHA titer had significant decrease and seroreversion in HIV positive patients (French et al., 2009).
However, another study found no association between HIV seropositivity and seroreversion of treponemal antibodies, in patients treated for early syphilis (Augenbraun et al., 1998). Also, seroreversion of treponemal antibodies had been reported in immunocompetent patients treated for early syphilis (Schroeter et al., 1972) or first episode of syphilis (Romanowski et al., 1991).

3.2 Post-HAART

Antiretroviral therapy significantly reduced the time to achieve response to syphilis treatment in HIV-positive patients (Gonzalez-Lopez et al., 2009).
Farhi et al. evaluated the effect of HIV on clinical and serologic features of syphilis at baseline and during follow-up in the pos-HAART era, in a retrospective cohort study of patients with syphilis treated according to the European guidelines. Serologic failure was defined as either a fourfold rise in VDRL titers 30-400 days after treatment or a lack of fourfold drop in VDRL titers at 270-400 days post treatment. Among 144 informative syphilis cases, a lower rate of serologic response was observed in HIV infected patients, however this difference was not significant (91.8% vs. 98.3%, p = 0.14). Also, a median delay to serologic response was similar in both group of patients (p = 0.44), HIV positive (117 days) and in HIV negative (123 days). Serologic failure was significantly associated with a history of previous syphilis (p < 0.05). The authors concluded that effect of HIV on serologic response to syphilis treatment is minimal or absent for patients under HAART treatment (Farhi et al., 2009; Farhi & Dupin, 2010). Another study evaluated whether the use of HAART impact syphilis serologic responses. Serologic failure was defined as the lack of fourfold decrease in RPR titers 9 - 12 months after therapy or a fourfold increase in titers a month or later after therapy. A total of 71 cases among 180 patients with syphilis presented serologic failure, and the median follow-up time was 5.3 years. CD4 cells count of < 200 cells/mL at the time of syphilis diagnosis was associated with an increased risk of serologic failure. The use of HAART was associated with 60% reduction in the rate of serologic failure, independent of concomitant CD4 cell response (Ghanem et al., 2008).

4. Neurosyphilis

Central neural system (CNS) involvements can occur during any stage of syphilis. CSF laboratory abnormalities are common in persons with early syphilis, even in the absence of clinical neurological findings. A CSF examination should be performed when clinical evidence of neurologic involvement is observed, including ocular manifestations frequently associated with neurosyphilis. There is no gold standard test to diagnose neurosyphilis. According to the diagnostic criteria, neurosyphilis can be defined in two categories, confirmed and presumptive, both can occur at any stage of syphilis. Confirmed neurosyphilis presents reactive CSF VDRL, while presumptive neurosyphilis is defined when patients present clinical signs or symptoms consistent with syphilis without an alternate diagnosis to account for these, non reactive CSF VDRL and CSF pleocytosis or elevated protein (Ghanem, 2010).

A positive VDRL results establishes a diagnosis of neurosyphilis, but negative VDRL does not exclude it. The use of CSF RPR is not currently recommended, because RPR is less specific in CSF. The CSF FTA-abs test is less specific than the VDRL for diagnosis of neurosyphilis, but it is highly sensitive. A negative CSF FTA-abs test excludes the diagnosis of neurosyphilis (Workowski & Berman, 2010).

An alternative CSF tests to diagnose neurosyphilis in HIV infected patients had been proposed when the CSF VDRL is nonreactive. The combination of the CSF FTA-abs and assessment of CSF B cells can be used to identify syphilis patients with and without neurosyphilis when the CSF VDRL is non reactive (Marra et al., 2004c).

According to the European guidelines, a patient should be treated as for neurosyphilis in the following conditions: reactive CSF VDRL and treponemal antibody tests (TP hemagglutination assay or FTA-abs), WBC-CSF exceeds $10/mm^3$ and IgG index is 0.70 or higher or the IgM index is 0.10 or higher in CSF (Goh & van Voorst Vader, 2001).

A study by Marra et al demonstrated that a serum RPR titer $\geq$ 1:32 is predictive of neurosyphilis in all patients with syphilis and that a peripheral blood CD4 cell count $\leq$ 350 cell/uL is an additional risk factor for neurosyphilis in HIV infected patients. Also, the risk associated with these parameters is independent of previous syphilis therapy and stage of syphilis (Marra et al., 2004a).

If CSF pleocytosis was present initially, a CSF examination should be repeated every 6 months until the cell count turn to normal (Workowski & Berman, 2010).

The success of therapy in patients with symptomatic neurosyphilis is assessed by resolution of symptoms and signs, and normalization of CSF abnormalities, including pleocytosis, elevated protein concentration or a reactive CSF VDRL test. If neurosyphilis is asymptomatic, normalization of CSF measures is the only means of assessing treatment success (Workowski & Berman, 2010). After therapy, the changes in CSF VDRL or CSF protein occur more slowly than cell counts, and persistent abnormalities might be less important. The leukocyte count is a sensitive measure of the effectiveness of therapy (Marra et al., 2000; Marra et al., 2004b).

Resolution of all serum and CSF abnormalities were resolved by 30 weeks in most patients not infected with HIV (Marra et al., 1996). Another study by the same group found that in most instances, normalization of serum RPR titer correctly predicts normalization of CSF and clinical measures after neurosyphilis treatment and follow-up lumbar puncture can be avoided. However, using the serum RPR criteria, 12-37% of individuals can be misclassified as experiencing treatment success, and among HIV infected patients, misclassification is most common in those not receiving anti-retroviral therapy (Marra et al., 2008). A study found that resolution of CSF abnormalities was slower in patients infected with HIV after treatment of neurosyphilis (Marra et al., 1996), particularly if the peripheral blood CD4 cells count is lower than 200 cell/uL (Marra et al., 2004c).

A study of neurosyphilis in a clinical cohort of HIV-1 infected patients found that HAART therapy to reverse immunosupression may help mitigate neurological complication of syphilis. In this cohort, the degree of immunosuppression, as measured by CD4 cell count, was an independent risk factor for developing neurosyphilis, and the use of HAART reduced the odds of neurosyphilis by 65%. Among patients diagnosed and treated for neurosyphilis, there was a trend for decreased risk of serological failure in patients who received six or more months of HAART therapy during a median follow-up of 4.3 years (Ghanem et al., 2008).

5. Syphilis during pregnancy and congenital syphilis

All women should be screened serologically for syphilis early in pregnancy. Serologic testing should be performed at 28-32 weeks' gestation and repeated at delivery. Also, any woman who delivers a stillborn infant after 20 weeks' gestation should be tested for syphilis. Serologic titers can be checked monthly in women at high risk for reinfection or in geographic areas in which the prevalence of syphilis is high. If serological screening was performed by treponemal antibody testing, pregnant with reactive results for treponemal antibodies should have confirmatory testing with nontreponemal tests with titers (Workowski & Berman, 2010).

Transplacental infection can occur at any stage pregnancy (Wicher & Wicher, 2001). Most cases of congenital syphilis occur as a result of a failure to detect and treat syphilis in pregnant women. The failure of treatment and congenital syphilis has been reported (Lasfargue et al., 2009; Marangoni et al., 2008).

Regardless of the regimen used to treat syphilis during pregnancy, clinicians should recognize the possibility of occasional treatment failures and the importance of adequate follow-up of infants at risk for congenital syphilis (Conover et al., 1998).

Factors that contribute to treatment failure include maternal stage of syphilis (early stage syphilis), advancing gestational age at treatment, higher VDRL titers at treatment and delivery, and a short interval from treatment to delivery, defined as ≤30 days, and these factors can be used to target neonates at high risk for congenital syphilis (Sheffield et al., 2002).

The diagnosis of congenital syphilis is based both, on a clinical evaluation and on laboratory investigations. Diagnosis is complicated because more than half of all infants are asymptomatic at birth, and sign in symptomatic infants may be subtle and nonspecific.

All infant born to women who have reactive serologic test for syphilis should be examined thoroughly for evidence for congenital syphilis, darkfield microscopy examination of suspicious lesions or body fluids also should be performed. Pathologic examination of the placenta or umbilical cord using specific fluorescent anti-treponemal antibody staining is suggested. Also, infants born to mothers who have reactive nontreponemal and treponemal test results should be evaluated with quantitative nontreponemal serological test (VDRL or RPR) performed on infant serum. It is not necessary to conduct a treponemal test on a newborn's serum, however a test to detect immunoglobulin IgM can be recommended (Workowski & Berman, 2010). The detection of specific IgM is currently the most sensitive serological method, and the presence of specific IgM should be considered as evidence of a congenital *T. pallidum* infection (Herremans et al., 2010).

In the past, a retrospective analysis of the serologic response to treatment of syphilis during pregnancy was performed. Treatment response was evaluated by comparing each post-treatment titer of a patient to her pre-treatment titer, and it was classified as a positive response (≥ fourfold titer decline) or a negative response (< fourfold titer decline). A

positive response following treatment was significant more likely if there was no prior history of syphilis or if there was a high initial RPR titer (> 32). Only 61% (33/54) had positive response at or greater than 3 months observations. The study revealed that an absence of a history of syphilis and an initial high RPR titer are predictive of a positive response following appropriate treatment (Galan et al., 1997).
Chang et al. performed a retrospective survey to determine the time of seroreversion of serological tests for syphilis in 52 uninfected newborn to mothers who were adequately treated for syphilis. Most seropositive untreated newborns became seronegative within 6 months after birth for the VDRL and within 1 year for the TPHA and FTAabs. However, 3 infants showed persistently positive VDRL and TPHA tests. The VDRL seroreversion were documented at 9 and 10 months after birth, and TPHA remained positive over 12 months. These infants had no clinical evidences of congenital syphilis and presented nonreactive 19S-IgM- FTAabs (Chang et al., 1995).
All seroreactive infants and infants whose mother were seroreactive at delivery should receive careful follow-up examinations and serologic nontreponemal test every 2-3 months Until the test become nonreactive or the titer has decreased fourfold. If the infant was adequately treated or was not infected, nontreponemal antibody titers should decline by age 3 months and should be nonreactive by age 6 months. The serologic response after therapy might be slower for infants treated after the neonatal period. (Workowski & Berman, 2010). Passively transferred maternal treponemal antibodies can be present in an infant until the age 15 months; therefore, a reactive treponemal test after age 18 months is diagnostic of congenital syphilis. Infants whose initial CSF evaluations are abnormal should undergo a repeat lumbar puncture approximately every 6 months until the results are normal (Workowski & Berman, 2010).

6. Potential markers

A specific anti-treponemal IgM-EIA may be helpful in monitoring the serological response to treatment in RPR/VDRL negative primary syphilis (French et al., 2009).
Recently, a study examined the relationship between neurosyphilis and CSF concentration of CXCL13 in HIV infected patients with syphilis. CXCL13 is a B cell chemoattractant chemokine (C-X-C motif) ligant 13. They found that, compared to patients with uncomplicated syphilis, CSF CXCL13 concentration is significantly higher in patients with both asymptomatic and symptomatic neurosyphilis, and CSF CXCL13 concentration declines after neurosyphilis treatment (Marra et al., 2010). This may be particularly useful marker for diagnosis and treatment response evaluation of neurosyphilis in HIV infected patients (Marra et al., 2010).

7. Conclusion

There is no direct microbiologic test of cure of syphilis disease. Treatment response in current practice can be defined clinically and/or serologically by regular follow-up of quantitative serologic test for nontreponemal antibody (VDRL or RPR). Also, it is difficult to distinguish relapse from reinfection. The specific IgM antibodies may be helpful in this issue. The most relevant markers of treatment response are essential to improve the follow-up accuracy. Current research should focus on stronger efficacy assessment tool than the actual nontreponemal serology in use. The search for direct *T. pallidum* identification methods such as exploring molecular marker by *T.pallidum* specific polymerase chain reaction may be a promising approach.

8. References

Agmon-Levin, N., Elbirt, D., Asher, I., Gradestein, S., Werner, B. & Sthoeger, Z. (2010). Syphilis and HIV co-infection in an Israeli HIV clinic: incidence and outcome. *International Journal of Std & Aids* Vol.21, No.4, (April 2010), pp. 249-252, ISSN 1758-1052

Anderson, J., Mindel, A., Tovey, S. J. & Williams, P. (1989). Primary and secondary syphilis, 20 years' experience. 3: Diagnosis, treatment, and follow up. *Genitourinary Medicine* Vol.65, No.4, (August 1989), pp. 239-243, ISSN 0266-4348

Augenbraun, M., Rolfs, R., Johnson, R., Joesoef, R. & Pope, V. (1998). Treponemal specific tests for the serodiagnosis of syphilis. Syphilis and HIV Study Group. *Sexually Transmitted Disease* Vol.25, No.10, (November 1998), pp. 549-552, ISSN 0148-5717

Brown, T. J., Yen-Moore, A. & Tyring, S. K. (1999). An overview of sexually transmitted diseases. Part I. *Journal of the American Academy of Dermatology* Vol.41, No.4, (October 1999), pp. 511-529, ISSN 0190-9622

Castro, R. R., Prieto, E. S., Santo, I., Azevedo, J. & Exposto, F. d. L. (2001). Evaluation of the Passive Particle Agglutination Test in the Serodiagnosis and Follow-up of Syphilis. *American Journal of Clinical Pathology* Vol.116, No.4, (October 2001), pp. 581-585, ISSN 1943-7722

Chang, S. N., Chung, K. Y., Lee, M. G. & Lee, J. B. (1995). Seroreversion of the serological tests for syphilis in the newborns born to treated syphilitic mothers. *Genitourinary Medicine* Vol.71, No.2, (April 1995), pp. 68-70, ISSN 0266-4348

Conover, C. S., Rend, C. A., Miller, G. B., Jr. & Schmid, G. P. (1998). Congenital syphilis after treatment of maternal syphilis with a penicillin regimen exceeding CDC guidelines. *Infectious diseases in obstetrics and gynecology* Vol.6, No.3, pp. 134-137, ISSN 1064-7449

Farhi, D., Benhaddou, N., Grange, P., Zizi, N., Deleuze, J., Morini, J. P., Gerhardt, P., Krivine, A., Avril, M. F. & Dupin, N. (2009). Clinical and serologic baseline and follow-up features of syphilis according to HIV status in the post-HAART era. *Medicine (Baltimore)* Vol.88, No.6, (November 2009), pp. 331-340, ISSN 1536-5964

Farhi, D. & Dupin, N. (2010). Management of syphilis in the HIV-infected patient: Facts and controversies. *Clinics in Dermatology* Vol.28, No.5, (August 2010), pp. 539-545, ISSN 0738-081X

Fiumara, N. J. (1977a). Treatment of secondary syphilis: an evaluation of 204 patients. *Sexually Transmitted Diseases* Vol.4, No.3, (July 1977), pp. 96-99, ISSN 0148-5717

Fiumara, N. J. (1977b). Treatment of seropositive primary syphilis: an evaluation of 196 patients. *Sexually Transmitted Diseases* Vol.4, No.3, (July 1977), pp. 92-95, ISSN 0148-5717

Fiumara, N. J. (1978). Treatment of early latent syphilis of less than a year's duration: an evaluation of 275 cases. *Sexually Transmitted Diseases* Vol.5, No.3, (Jul 1978), pp. 85-88, ISSN 0148-5717

Fiumara, N. J. (1979). Serologic responses to treatment of 128 patients with late latent syphilis. *Sexually Transmitted Diseases* Vol.6, No.4, (October 1979), pp. 243-246, ISSN 0148-5717

Fraser, C. M., Norris, S. J., Weinstock, G. M., White, O., Sutton, G. G., Dodson, R., Gwinn, M., Hickey, E. K., Clayton, R., Ketchum, K. A., Sodergren, E., Hardham, J. M., McLeod, M. P., Salzberg, S., Peterson, J., Khalak, H., Richardson, D., Howell, J. K., Chidambaram, M., Utterback, T., McDonald, L., Artiach, P., Bowman, C., Cotton, M. D., Fujii, C., Garland, S., Hatch, B., Horst, K., Roberts, K., Sandusky, M.,

Weidman, J., Smith, H. O. & Venter, J. C. (1998). Complete Genome Sequence of Treponema pallidum, the Syphilis Spirochete. *Science* Vol.281, No.5375, (July 1998), pp. 375-388, ISSN 0036-8075

French, P., Gomberg, M., Janier, M., Schmidt, B., van Voorst Vader, P. & Young, H. (2009). IUSTI: 2008 European Guidelines on the Management of Syphilis. *International Journal of Std & Aids* Vol.20, No.5, (May 2009), pp. 300-309, ISSN 0956-4624

Galan, H. L., Montalvo, J. F. & Deaver, J. (1997). Retrospective analysis of the serologic response to the treatment of syphilis during pregnancy. *Infectious diseases in obstetrics and gynecology* Vol.5, No.1, pp. 23-28, ISSN 1064-7449

Ghanem, K. G. (2010). Neurosyphilis: A Historical Perspective and Review. *CNS Neuroscience & Therapeutics* Vol.16, No.5, (July 2010), pp. e157-e168, ISSN 1755-5949

Ghanem, K. G., Erbelding, E. J., Wiener, Z. S. & Rompalo, A. M. (2007). Serological response to syphilis treatment in HIV-positive and HIV-negative patients attending sexually transmitted diseases clinics. *Sexually Transmitted Infections* Vol.83, No.2, (April 2007), pp. 97-101, ISSN 1368-4973

Ghanem, K. G., Moore, R. D., Rompalo, A. M., Erbelding, E. J., Zenilman, J. M. & Gebo, K. A. (2008). Antiretroviral Therapy Is Associated with Reduced Serologic Failure Rates for Syphilis among HIV-Infected Patients. *Clinical Infectious Diseases* Vol.47, No.2, (July 2008), pp. 258-265, ISSN 1537-6591

Goh, B. T. & van Voorst Vader, P. C. (2001). European guideline for the management of syphilis. *International Journal of STD & AIDS* Vol.12, No.suppl_2, (October 2001), pp. 14-26, ISSN 0956-4624

Gonzalez-Lopez, J. J., Guerrero, M. L., Lujan, R., Tostado, S. F., de Gorgolas, M. & Requena, L. (2009). Factors determining serologic response to treatment in patients with syphilis. *Clinical Infectious Diseases* Vol.49, No.10, (November 2009), pp. 1505-1511, ISSN 1537-6591

Haas, J. S., Bolan, G., Larsen, S. A., Clement, M. J., Bacchetti, P. & Moss, A. R. (1990). Sensitivity of Treponemal Tests for Detecting Prior Treated Syphilis during Human Immunodeficiency Virus Infection. *Journal of Infectious Diseases* Vol.162, No.4, (October 1990), pp. 862-866, ISSN 1537-6613

Herremans, T., Kortbeek, L. & Notermans, D. W. (2010). A review of diagnostic tests for congenital syphilis in newborns. *European journal of clinical microbiology & infectious diseases* Vol.29, No.5, (May 2010), pp. 495-501, ISSN 1435-4373

Horberg, M. A., Ranatunga, D. K., Quesenberry, C. P., Klein, D. B. & Silverberg, M. J. (2010). Syphilis Epidemiology and Clinical Outcomes in HIV-Infected and HIV-Uninfected Patients in Kaiser Permanente Northern California. *Sexually Transmitted Diseases* Vol.37, No.1, (January 2010), pp. 53-58 ISSN 0148-5717

Johnson, P. D., Graves, S. R., Stewart, L., Warren, R., Dwyer, B. & Lucas, C. R. (1991). Specific syphilis serological tests may become negative in HIV infection. *Aids* Vol.5, No.4, (April 1991), pp. 419-423, ISSN 0269-9370

Kim, D. K., Lee, M. G. & Lee, J. B. (1989). Changes of serum IgG antibody reactivity to protein antigens of Treponema pallidum in syphilis patients after treatment. *Journal of Korean Medical Science* Vol.4, No.2, (June 1989), pp. 63-69, ISSN 1598-6357

Kofoed, K., Gerstoft, J., Mathiesen, L. R. & Benfield, T. (2006). Syphilis and Human Immunodeficiency Virus (HIV)-1 Coinfection: Influence on CD4 T-Cell Count, HIV-1 Viral Load, and Treatment Response. *Sexually Transmitted Diseases* Vol.33, No.3, (March 2006), pp. 143-148, ISSN 0148-5717

Lasfargue, M., Thummler, S., Perelman, S. & de Ricaud, D. (2009). Congenital syphilis: a case report. *Archives de Pédiatrie* Vol.16 No.Suppl 2, (October 2009), pp. S123-126, ISSN 1769-664X

Luger, A., Schmidt, B. & Spendlingwimmer, I. (1977). Quantitative evaluation of the FTA-ABS-IgM and VDRL test in treated and untreated syphilis. *The British Journal of Venereal Diseases* Vol.53, No.5, (October 1977), pp. 287-291, ISSN 0007-134X

Malone, J. L., Wallace, M. R., Hendrick, B. B., LaRocco, A., Tonon, E., Brodine, S. K., Bowler, W. A., Lavin, B. S., Hawkins, R. E. & Oldfield, E. C. (1995). Syphilis and neurosyphilis in a human immunodeficiency virus type-1 seropositive population: Evidence for frequent serologic relapse after therapy. *The American Journal of Medicine* Vol.99, No.1, (July 1995), pp. 55-63, ISSN 1555-7162

Manavi, K. & McMillan, A. (2007). The outcome of treatment of early latent syphilis and syphilis with undetermined duration in HIV-infected and HIV-uninfected patients. *International Journal of Std & Aids* Vol.18, No.12, (December 2007), pp. 814-818, ISSN 0956-4624

Marangoni, A., Moroni, A., Tridapalli, E., Capretti, M. G., Farneti, G., Faldella, G., D'Antuono, A. & Cevenini, R. (2008). Antenatal syphilis serology in pregnant women and follow-up of their infants in northern Italy. *Clinical Microbiology Infection* Vol.14, No.11, (November 2008), pp. 1065-1068, ISSN 1469-0691

Marra, C. M., Boutin, P., McArthur, J. C., Hurwitz, S., Simpson, P. A., Haslett, J. A., van der Horst, C., Nevin, T. & Hook, E. W., 3rd (2000). A pilot study evaluating ceftriaxone and penicillin G as treatment agents for neurosyphilis in human immunodeficiency virus-infected individuals. *Clinical Infectious Diseases* Vol.30, No.3, (March 2000), pp. 540-544, ISSN 1058-4838

Marra, C. M., Longstreth, W. T., Jr., Maxwell, C. L. & Lukehart, S. A. (1996). Resolution of serum and cerebrospinal fluid abnormalities after treatment of neurosyphilis. Influence of concomitant human immunodeficiency virus infection. *Sexually Transmitted Diseases* Vol.23, No.3, (May 1996), pp. 184-189, ISSN 0148-5717

Marra, C. M., Maxwell, C. L., Smith, S. L., Lukehart, S. A., Rompalo, A. M., Eaton, M., Stoner, B. P., Augenbraun, M., Barker, D. E., Corbett, J. J., Zajackowski, M., Raines, C., Nerad, J., Kee, R. & Barnett, S. H. (2004a). Cerebrospinal fluid abnormalities in patients with syphilis: association with clinical and laboratory features. *The Journal of Infectious Diseases* Vol.189, No.3, (February 2004), pp. 369-376, ISSN 0022-1899

Marra, C. M., Maxwell, C. L., Tantalo, L., Eaton, M., Rompalo, A. M., Raines, C., Stoner, B. P., Corbett, J. J., Augenbraun, M., Zajackowski, M., Kee, R. & Lukehart, S. A. (2004b). Normalization of cerebrospinal fluid abnormalities after neurosyphilis therapy: does HIV status matter? *Clinical Infectious Diseases* Vol.38, No.7, (April 2004), pp. 1001-1006, ISSN 1537-6591

Marra, C. M., Maxwell, C. L., Tantalo, L. C., Sahi, S. K. & Lukehart, S. A. (2008). Normalization of serum rapid plasma reagin titer predicts normalization of cerebrospinal fluid and clinical abnormalities after treatment of neurosyphilis. *Clinical Infectious Diseases* Vol.47, No.7, (October 2008), pp. 893-899, ISSN 1537-6591

Marra, C. M., Tantalo, L. C., Maxwell, C. L., Dougherty, K. & Wood, B. (2004c). Alternative cerebrospinal fluid tests to diagnose neurosyphilis in HIV-infected individuals. *Neurology* Vol.63, No.1, (July 2004), pp. 85-88, ISSN 1526-632X

Marra, C. M., Tantalo, L. C., Sahi, S. K., Maxwell, C. L. & Lukehart, S. A. (2010). CXCL13 as a cerebrospinal fluid marker for neurosyphilis in HIV-infected patients with syphilis. *Sexually Transmitted Diseases* Vol.37, No.5, (May 2010), pp. 283-287, ISSN 1537-4521

McMillan, A. & Young, H. (2008). Reactivity in the Venereal Diseases Research Laboratory test and the Mercia(R) IgM enzyme immunoassay after treatment of early syphilis. *International Journal of Std & Aids* Vol.19, No.10, (October 2008), pp. 689-693, ISSN 0956-4624

Palmer, H. M., Higgins, S. P., Herring, A. J. & Kingston, M. A. (2003). Use of PCR in the diagnosis of early syphilis in the United Kingdom. *Sexually Transmitted Infectious* Vol.79, No.6, (December 2003), pp. 479-483, ISSN 1368-4973

Romanowski, B., Forsey, E., Prasad, E., Lukehart, S., Tam, M. & Hook, E. W., 3rd (1987). Detection of Treponema pallidum by a fluorescent monoclonal antibody test. *Sexually Transmitted Diseases* Vol.14, No.3, (July 1987), pp. 156-159, ISSN 0148-5717

Romanowski, B., Sutherland, R., Fick, G. H., Mooney, D. & Love, E. J. (1991). Serologic response to treatment of infectious syphilis. *Annals Internal Medicine* Vol.114, No.12, (June 1991), pp. 1005-1009, ISSN 0003-4819

Rotty, J., Anderson, D., Garcia, M., Diaz, J., Van de Waarsenburg, S., Howard, T., Dennison, A., Lewin, S. R., Elliott, J. H. & Hoy, J. (2010). Preliminary assessment of Treponema pallidum-specific IgM antibody detection and a new rapid point-of-care assay for the diagnosis of syphilis in human immunodeficiency virus-1-infected patients. *International Journal of Std & Aids* Vol.21, No.11, (November 2010), pp. 758-764, ISSN 1758-1052

Schmidt, B. L., Luger, A., Duschet, P., Seifert, W. & Gschnait, F. (1994). Specific IgM tests in syphilis diagnosis. *Hautarzt* Vol.45, No.10, (October 1994), pp. 685-689, ISSN 0017-8470

Schroeter, A. L., Lucas, J. B., Price, E. V. & Falcone, V. H. (1972). Treatment for early syphilis and reactivity of serologic tests. *Jama* Vol.221, No.5, (July 31), pp. 471-476, ISSN 0098-7484

Sheffield, J. S., Sanchez, P. J., Wendel, G. D., Fong, D. W. I., Margraf, L. R., Zeray, F., McIntire, D. D. & Rogers, B. B. (2002). Placental histopathology of congenital syphilis. *Obstetrics and Gynecology* Vol.100, No.1, (July 2002), pp. 126-133, ISSN 0029-7844

Singh, A. E. & Romanowski, B. (1999). Syphilis: Review with emphasis on clinical, epidemiologic, and some biologic features. *Clinical Microbiology Reviews* Vol.12, No.2, (April 1999), pp. 187-209, ISSN 0893-8512

Talwar, S., Tutakne, M. A. & Tiwari, V. D. (1992). VDRL titres in early syphilis before and after treatment. *Genitourinary Medicine* Vol.68, No.2, (April 1992), pp. 120-122, ISSN 0266-4348

Telzak, E. E., Greenberg, M. S., Harrison, J., Stoneburner, R. L. & Schultz, S. (1991). Syphilis treatment response in HIV-infected individuals. *Aids* Vol.5, No.5, (May 1991), pp. 591-595, ISSN 0269-9370

Walter, T., Lebouche, B., Miailhes, P., Cotte, L., Roure, C., Schlienger, I. & Trepo, C. (2006). Symptomatic Relapse of Neurologic Syphilis after Benzathine Penicillin G Therapy for Primary or Secondary Syphilis in HIV-Infected Patients. *Clinical Infectious Diseases* Vol.43, No.6, (September 2006), pp. 787-790, ISSN 1537-6591

Wicher, V. & Wicher, K. (2001). Pathogenesis of maternal-fetal syphilis revisited. *Clinical Infectious Diseases* Vol.33, No.3, (August 2001), pp. 354-363, ISSN 1058-4838

Workowski, K. A. & Berman, S. (2010). Sexually Transmitted Diseases Guidelines, 2010. *Morbity and Mortality Weekly report* Vol.59, No.RR12, (December 2010), pp. 26-40, ISSN 1545-8601

Yinnon, A. M., Coury-Doniger, P., Polito, R. & Reichman, R. C. (1996). Serologic Response to Treatment of Syphilis in Patients With HIV Infection. *Archives Internal Medicine* Vol.156, No.3, (February 1996), pp. 321-325, ISSN 0003-9926

8

Syphilis and Blood Safety in Developing Countries

Claude Tayou Tagny
Faculty of Medicine and Biomedical Sciences, University of Yaoundé I
Cameroon

1. Introduction

Syphilis is still a public health problem in the world. The World Health Organization estimated that approximately 12 million new cases are reported each year in the world with more than 90 percent from developing countries (Centers for Disease Control [CDC], 2007; World Health Organization [WHO], 2001). Moreover, syphilis has acquired a higher potential of morbidity and mortality with the increasing prevalence of HIV infection. If syphilis is rare in developed countries, it is much more common in developing countries where prevalence can reach 25% amongst blood donors (Tagny & al., 2009, 2010).The infection is transmitted from person to person through contact with a syphilis ulcer (during vaginal, anal, or oral sex). An infected mother can infect her fetus via the placenta. Furthermore, intravenous drug addicts or other infected person can transmit syphilis through infected blood products i.e. through blood transfusion or use of infected needles for example (Workowski & Berman, 2006).

2. Transfusion transmissibility of syphilis

Fordyce reported the first case of transfusion-transmitted syphilis in 1915. More than 100 cases have subsequently been reported in different countries including USA and Great Britain (CDC, 2004; Henneberg M. & Henneberg R.J., 1994; Lobdell & al., 1974). However, the numbers of transfusion-transmitted syphilis cases has decreased all over the world. In the past 35 years, only three cases of transfusion-transmitted syphilis have been reported in the English literature and the last one was reported since more than forty years ago in USA (Brant & al., 2007; CDC, 2004; Chambers & al., 1969; Hook & Peeling, 2004). The absence of transfusion-transmitted syphilis in many developed countries leads to question the rationale for continuing syphilis testing of blood donors.

Syphilis is a transfusion-transmitted infection (TTI) due to a spirocheta called *Treponema pallidum*. The germ is present in the blood of a contaminated blood donor and infects the recipient. The transmissibility of syphilis by blood transfusion has been frequently reported, chiefly based on animal experiments. Cases of syphilis transmitted by blood have been described in literature, with more than a hundred cases since the first description. The main cases reported were shown to occur when donors were in the primary or secondary stage of the disease. (Gardella & al., 2002; Orton, 2001; Risseeuw-Appel & Kothe, 1983; Singh & Romanowski, 1999; Soendjojo & al., 1982). *T. pallidum* may be found in the blood stream, but

levels are variable, and bacteremia is often short-lived even in recent contamination. Moreover, the treponemes are relatively fragile and sensitive to cold; storage below +20°c for more than 72 hours destroys the organism and reduces dramatically the infectious risk. Although clearly potentially infectious, the risk of transmission through the transfusion of blood and blood components stored below +20°c is very low (Orton, 2001; Wendel, 1994). Platelet concentrates usually stored at a temperature above +20°C or blood directly transfused few hours after collection comprises a higher risk of transmitting syphilis. This is the case in many developing countries with limited blood supply where blood is collected from family donors and frequently transfused in the following hours or days. Thus, the screening test is considered essential as most blood transfusion services are concerned by storage of blood products stored either above +20°C or not stored below +20°C for more than 4 days. Furthermore, it is actually shown that the deferral of blood products screened positive also reduces the risk of contamination from HIV and HBV.
When the germ is transmitted to the recipient, some signs appear a few weeks later notably macular lesions on the palms, headache, arthralgia, fever, headache, peripheral lymphs nodes and more rarely jaundice. For all the reported cases, there was neither a history of venereal disease nor presence of sores on the blood donor at the time of donation. However, many cases were associated with appearance of a sore on the blood donor few days after the donation. Thus, syphilis can be transmitted from donors who are clinically and biologically negative. It is clear that medical selection and mainly information and questionning are essential to identify those who have been exposed to infection during the preceding two months.
Some other diseases are caused by other species or subspecies of Treponema: Yaws (*Treponema pertenue*), Pinta (*Treponema carateum*) and Bejel (*Treponema endemicum*). Yaws and pinta may potentially be transmitted by transfusion, but few data is available. Bejel is unlikely to be transmitted and infect individuals (Chambers & al., 1969; Wendel, 1994). These diseases usually have clear symptoms that would lead to donor deferral.
Strategies of safety were proposed and modified during the years until the adoption in 1987 by the WHO of a common international strategy. Several steps and strategies were elaborated as well by the international organizations (WHO, the International Society of Blood Transfusion, the American Association of Blood Banks) and the blood banks. Their general recommendations focus on the control of the bacterial dissemination of the disease through blood transfusion by the selection of low risk blood donors and the screening of the disease by efficient lab tests. The strategies of reduction of this risk of transfusion transmissible infections associates the natural medical selection the effective biological qualification, the reduction of pathogens by a physico-chemical treatment of the products and the rational use of the prepared products. However, blood safety begins by the implementation of organized blood centres, of a quality system, hemovigilance, and application of safety measures in transfusion. The organization of blood centres is related to the implementation of blood supply programs and blood safety strategies by a well-organized centre, national or regional. Blood banks are frequently used as a base of transfusion. A Quality system includes management, training, norms, documentation traceability and evaluation. Haemovigilance is defined as a set of organized surveillance procedures relating to adverse or unexpected events or reactions in donors or recipients. In the transfusion chain, the first to be considered is the safe blood donor.

3. Syphilis and blood donor

Blood donors with high-risk sexual behaviour and other risk factors may be infected by syphilis and compromise the safety of blood used for transfusion. The medical selection of the blood donors consists of information of the donor, the finding of the risk factors in the behaviours and the medical history using a questionnaire, the physical examination in order to find clinical signs of the infection. Donor deferral follows identification of any risk. Medical selection is crucial because it could permit to defer more than half of infected donors, especially the ones in the early period of infection here laboratory tests are not efficient (de Almeida Neto & al, 2007; Tagny, 2009).

In some European countries, the prevalence of *T. pallidum* infection in the general population and thus in blood donors has been increasing since last two decades. An increase in syphilis infections has been associated to the high incidence of HIV. Moreover, an infected blood donor with syphilis is more than 5 times more likely to be HIV-positive. However, the prevalence of syphilis is still very low in developed countries and the very rare cases of recipient contamination raised the question of whether syphilis screening was still necessary for blood donors. In developing countries, the prevalence of positive serologic tests for syphilis can reach 25%. The prevalence is however very variable from one area to another and from a country to another. In such settings, the poor quality of laboratory screening due to the lack of equipment, training personnel, reagents and standard procedures highlights the need of the systematic and better screening for syphilis to help ensure a safer blood supply. Very little systematic information is available on the profile of positive blood donors including differences between donors with recent versus past infection. The exclusion of donors with past and treated infection is still a matter of discussion. Abusive exclusion reduces the blood supply and could be problematic in developing countries. However, past history of syphilis may be high-risk sexual behaviour associated to transmitted transfusion infection such as syphilis itself and HIV. The transfusion risk of syphilis is closely related to risk factors in the blood donor, in particular the sexual behaviours, the disease being primarily transmitted by sexual route. The rates of infection are highest amongst homosexual (gay) men - or men who have sex with men (Vall-Mayans & al, 2006). Recent syphilis infections have been shown to be associated with younger age, male-male sex, two or more sex partners, past syphilis treatment, past syphilis history, HIV seropositivity. Risk factors usually associated with transfusion transmitted syphillis also include more than one sexual partner, prostitution, bisexuality (men having sex with both men and women), intravenous drug use, and skin scarification (tattoing,blood rituals).

In developing countries, most blood donors infected are first-time donors. The prevalence of syphilis is one of the highest amongst the TTI screened in developing countries. The problem of this disease, first of all, is its high prevalence in blood donors in various areas of Africa. The recent prevalence were 3.7 % in Congo (Batina & al 2007), 7.9 % in Ghana (Adjei & al., 2003; Ampofo & al., 2002) and 9.1 % in Cameroon (Mbanya & al., 2003; Tagny & al., 2009). It is just as high in females as in males, in the different age groups and in voluntary donor as well as family donors. The family blood donation and remunerated blood donation, mostly found in developing countries is statiscally associated with higher prevalence of the disease (Batina & al., 2007; Tagny & al., 2010). The donors who have been positive for syphilis during the previous donation are less likely to donate again, whereas donors who were negative for the presence of syphilis in the past would be more likely to donate again. In countries, which use a medical questionnaire for selection of blood donor, there are usually questions related to infection with syphilis. These questions concentrate particularly on sexual behavior (a number of sexual partners, use of condoms, past history of sexually transmitted diseases) and sometimes on specific symptoms observed during clinical examination. However, medical selection remains ineffective for several reasons:

- Difficulty of understanding the questions due to the level of education (ignorance of the transmissible infections by blood transfusion) (Nébié & al., 2007; Agbovi & al., 2006), linguistic and cultural (taboos) barriers;
- Discrete expression of the disease in its primary phase. The syphilitic rosella is not clearly visible on dark skin.
- Suppression of clinical signs and symptoms by the various antibiotics following self - medication (ampicilline, penicillin). Thus, the biological screening of this disease remains essential to defer blood donors at risk.

Identified safe donors must be retained in the pool of repeated donors and frequently informed and educated to avoid risky behaviours.

4. Syphilis and screening of blood donation

Serological tests for syphilis contributed greatly to the detection of *T. pallidum* infection in blood donors and especially in those who were not identified during the medical selection. Wasserman (Henneberg M. & Henneberg R.J., 1994; Rose & al., 1997) developed the first test of syphilis in 1906. Although it had some false positive results, it was a major advancement in the prevention of syphilis because it helped to diagnose the disease before the clinical manifestation and thus prevent its spread. In the 1930s the Hinton test, developed by William Augustus Hinton, and based on flocculation, was shown to be more specific than the Wassermann test. At the beginning of the 20th century newer tests were developed. Present-day, several labs tests, treponemic or not treponemic exist, among which rapid tests, immunological tests, and genomic (Young & al., 2000). Neither there is a specific type of method absolutely indicated, nor is there any confirmatory algorithm for testing based on the different assays available. In fact, the laboratory assessment of syphilis is generally based on the detection of antibodies against *T. pallidum* antigens in blood by the use of either specific or nonspecific reagents. The detection of genomic particle are more specific but not affordable for most of laboratories (Marfin & al., 2001; Orton & al. 2002).

The detection of specific Treponema antigens is possible using methods as passive agglutination, as *T. pallidum* hemagglutination (TPHA) assay or the *T. pallidum* particle agglutination (TPPA) assay, indirect immunofluorescence as the fluorescent treponemal antibody absorbed (FTA-ABS) assay or enzyme immunoassay (EIA) for the detection of specific IgG and IgM or total Ig. Non-treponemal methods are based on non-treponemal lipid antigens (cardiolipin), using frequently the flocculation technique. Of these, the Venereal Disease Research Laboratory (VDRL) and rapid plasma reagin (RPR) tests are the most commonly used. These tests are cheap, fast and more sensitive (Montoya & al. 2006; WHO, 2006). They are able to identify the contaminated blood donors few days before the treponemal test and thus useful for acute infection. However, VDRL and RPR cannot be automated and are time-consuming if used for large scale testing. Moreover, they produce more false positive results. These tests are routinely used to screen blood donors. False positives on the rapid tests can be seen in viral infections such as hepatitis, tuberculosis, malaria, or varicella. Thus, non-treponemal tests should be followed up when possible by a treponemal test. The treponemal tests are based on monoclonal antibodies and immunofluorescence; they are more specific and more expensive. The tests based on enzyme-linked immunoassays are the more specific and are usually used to confirm the results of simpler screening tests for syphilis. According to the guidelines published by the U.S. Centers for Disease Control and Prevention, the diagnosis of syphilis should be based on the results of at least two tests: one treponemal and the other non treponemal (CDC, 2006; CDC, 2004). According to WHO, blood banks may choose Venereal Disease Research Laboratory (VDRL), rapid plasma reagin (RPR), or enzyme immunoassay (EIA). VDRL and RPR are sensitive for recent syphilis infection, but not for past infection. Screening should be performed using a highly sensitive and specific test for treponemal antibodies: either TPHA or enzyme immunoassay. In populations where there is a high incidence of syphilis, screening should be performed using a non-treponemal assay: VDRL or RPR. EIA can detect past or recent infection, but may result in rejecting non-infectious blood with distant past infection (Cole & al., 2007). However, one should remember that the reliability of the screening and the diagnosis include the performances as well as the quality assessment notably the use of standard operating procedures, norms, training of the personnel and management of quality.

The screening for syphilis is frequently carried out on the African blood donor, and national policies often include the disease in the list of ITT to be screened at the time of blood donation. More than 90 % of blood collected in Africa in the year 2004 was screened for syphilis (Tapko & al., 2005). The techniques used for screening are different from one country to another: VDRL or RPR alone for some, VDRL + TPHA for others (Tagny, 2009). Developing countries are characterized by a difficult epidemiologic, sociological and economic environment which limits the implementation of a high quality of blood safety. Thus, this context requires that tests and algorithms should be selected so that they correspond with the high prevalence of the disease, limited technical know-how of the personnel and limited availability of reagents and equipments. The selection criteria of screening strategy must include simple techniques, reliability, sustainability and cost effectiveness. Regular supply of electricity, freezer and ELISA kits is mostly found in big cities and barely available in small towns. Several blood banks use rapid test technique as it does not required sophisticated lab materials (Tagny & al., 2009). Screening strategies must also take into account the training of technicians, guarantee their capacity to carry out the test and provide reliable results.

5. Other blood safety issues

The good clinical use of the blood products is an essential stage of blood safety with respect to syphilis. It relates to the definition and the respect of the indications of transfusion, but also recording, analysis and diffusion of adverse reactions due to the infection. Each blood bank or transfusion service (national or regional) is responsible for ensuring blood safety to their patients. They should minimize unnecessary transfusions by prevention of conditions that result in the need for transfusion, reduce blood loss by using good surgical and anaesthetic techniques, or use simple alternatives for volume replacement. These strategies could be done with the help of organisations such as transfusion committees in each hospital, national committee on the clinical use of blood, and a national haemovigilance system.

Blood safety also consists of the use of physico-chemical treatment (filter on blood bag, use of amotosalen or ribavirin). This treatment of donated blood has shown its capacity to reduce the transmissibility of many germs especially in plasma and platelets. Once inside the pathogen, amotosalen or ribavirin docks in between the nucleic acid base pairs and blocks irreversibly the replication of DNA and ARN, thus preventing the proliferation. The physico-chemical treatment cannot be used on erythrocytes and are costly, thus less suitable for resources limited countries where whole blood and red blood cell concentrates are mostly used.

6. Conclusion

The challenge and perspectives of syphilis during transfusion is related to improvement of clinical selection of blood donor (identifying the precise risk factors) and to development of tools for the treatment of red blood cell concentrates. Syphills was the first infectious agent shown to be transmitted by blood transfusion and, in the past, there was a reasonably significant number of transmissions. Occasional cases still occur even today in some countries with a high incidence of syphillis. However, it is very unlikely that transfusion has ever been a major factor in the spread of the disease. In low incidence countries, the vast majority of cases of syphillis identified in blood donors are due to old infections that have been treated succesfully and present no risk of transfusion transmission. With the exclusion of high risk donors, screening for *T. pallidum* and storage of most blood components at or below +4°C before transfusion, makes the risk of post transfusion syphilis almost negligible in many countries. The challenges and the perspectives of the disease during transfusion are related to improvement clinical selection of blood donor (identifying the precise risk factors) and to the development of tools for treatment of red blood cell concentrates.

Prevention of the spread of syphillis is primarily by education and developpement of effective and treatment programmes. All patients with syphilis should be tested for HIV. Sexually transmitted diseases in general are the major route of infection while transfusion is only a minor route. Eliminating high risk sexual behaviours is very effective in helping prevent Syphilis. Proper and consistent use of a latex condom can also reduce the spread of syphilis. Moreover, donors sexually exposed to a person with primary, secondary, or early latent syphilis within 90 days preceding the diagnosis should be assumed to be infected. They should be treated and educated, even if they are seronegative at the time of donation.

7. References

Adjei, A.A.; Kudzi, W.; Armah, H.; Adiku, T.; Amoah, AG. & Ansah, J. (2003). Prevalence of antibodies to syphilis among blood donors in Accra Ghana. *Jpn J Infect Dis*, Vol 56, N°4, pp.165–7.

Agbovi, K.K.; Kolou, M.; Fétéké, L.; Haudrechy, D.; North, M.L. & Ségbéna, A.Y. (2006). Etude des connaissances, attitudes et pratiques en matière de don de sang. Enquête sociologique dans la population de Lomé (Togo). *Transfus Clin Biol* Vol 13, pp.260–5.

Ampofo, W.; Nii-Trebi, N.; Ansah, J.; Abe, K.; Naito, H.; Aidoo, S.; Nuvor, V.; Brandful, J.; Yamamoto, N.; Ofori-Adjei, D. & Ishikawa, K. (2002). Prevalence of blood-borne infectious diseases in blood donors in Ghana. *J Clin Microbiol.*, Vol 40, pp.3523–3525.

Batina, A.; Kabemba, S. & Malengela, R. (2007).Infectious markers among blood donors in Democratic Republic of Congo (DRC) *Revue Médicale de Bruxelles,* Vol 28, N°3, pp 145–9.

Brant, L.J.; Bukasa, A.; Davison, K.L.; Newham, J. & Barbara, J.A. (2007). Increase in recently acquired syphilis infections in English, Welsh and Northern Irish blood donors. *Vox Sang.* Vol 93, pp.19–26.

Centers for Disease Control (CDC) (2004). STD Facts - Syphilis. Centers for Disease Control. Retrieved on 2007-05-30.

Centers for Disease Control (2006). "Sexually Transmitted Diseases Treatment Guidelines, 2006". MMWR 55 (RR-11): 24-32.

Chambers, R.W., Foley, H.T., Schmidt, P.J. (1969). Transmission of syphilis by fresh blood components. Transfusion, Vol 9, pp. 32–34.

Cole, M.J.; Perry, K.R. & Parry, J.V. (2007). Comparative evaluation of 15 serological assays for the detection of syphilis infection. *Eur J Clin Microbiol Infect Dis,* Vol 26, N°10, pp. 705–13.

de Almeida Neto, C. ; McFarland, W. ; Murphy, E.L. ; Chen, S. & Nogueira, F.A. (2007). Risk factors for human immunodeficiency virus infection among blood donors in Sao Paulo, Brazil, and their relevance to current donor deferral criteria. *Transfusion.* Vol 47, pp. 608–614.

Gardella, C.; Marfin, A.A.; Kahn, R.H.; Swint, E. & Markowitz, L.E.(2002). Persons with early syphilis identified through blood or plasma donation screening in the United States. *J Infect Dis.* Vol 185,pp.545–549.

Lobdell, J. & Owsley, D. (1974). "The origin of syphilis". *Journal of Sex Research* Vol 10, N°1, pp. 76-79.

Henneberg, M. & Henneberg, R.J. (1994). Treponematosis in an Ancient Greek colony of Metaponto, Southern Italy 580-250 BCE in *The Origin of Syphilis in Europe, Before or After 1493?* Centre Archeologique du Var, Editions Errance, pp. 92-98.

Hook, E.W. & Peeling, R.W. (2004). Syphilis control—continuing challenge. *N Engl J Med.* Vol.351, pp.122–124.

Marfin, A.A.; Liu, H.; Sutton, M.Y.; Steiner, B.; Pillay, A. & Markowitz, L.E.(2001). Amplification of the DNA polymerase I gene of *Treponema pallidum* from whole blood of persons with syphilis. *Diagn Microbiol Infect Dis.* Vol. 40, pp. 163–166.

Mbanya, D.N.; Takam, D. & Ndumbe, P.M.(2003). Serological findings amongst first time blood donors in Yaoundé´. Cameroon: is safe donation a reality or a myth? *Transfus Med,* Vol.13, N°5, pp.267–73.

Montoya, J.P.; Lukehart, S.A.; Brentlinger, P.E.; Blanco, A.J.; Floriano, F.: Sairosse, J. et al.(2006). Comparison of the diagnostic accuracy of a rapid immunochromatographic test and the rapid plasma reagin test for antenatal syphilis screening in Mozambique. *Bull World Health Organ,* Vol.84, pp.97–104.

Nébié, K.Y. ; Olinger, C.M. ; Kafando, E. ; Dahourou, H. ; Diallo, S. ; Kientega, Y., et al. Faible niveau de connaissances des donneurs de sang au Burkina Faso; une entrave potentielle à la sécurité transfusionnelle. *Transfus Clin Biol,* Vol. 14, pp.446–52.

Orton, S.L.; Liu, H.; Dodd, R.Y. & Williams, A.E. (2002). Prevalence of circulating *Treponema pallidum* DNA and RNA in blood donors with confirmed-positive syphilis tests. *Transfusion,* Vol.42, pp.94–99.

Orton, S. (2001).Syphilis and blood donors: what we know, what we do not know, and what we need to know. *Transfus Med Rev.* Vol.15, pp.282–291.

Risseuw-Appel, I.M. & Kothe, F.C. (1983).Transfusion syphilis: a case report. *Sex Transm Dis.* Vol.10, pp.200–201.

Rose, M. (1997). "Origins of Syphilis". *Archaeology* Vol.50, N°1, pp. 23-56.

Singh, A.E. & Romanowski, B. (1999). Syphilis: review with emphasis on clinical, epidemiologic, and some biologic features. *Clin. Microbiol. Rev,*Vol. 12, pp.187-209.

Soendjojo, A.; Boedisantoso, M.; Ilias, M.I. & Rahardjo, D.(1982). Syphilis d'emblée due to blood transfusion. Case report. *Br J Vener Dis.* Vol.58, pp.149–150.

Tagny, C.T. ; Diarra, A. ; Yahaya, R. ; Hakizimana, M. ; Nguessan, A. ; Mbensa, G., et al. Characteristics of blood donors and donated blood in Sub-Saharan Francophone Africa. (2009).*Transfusion,* Vol. 49, pp.1592-9.

Tagny, C.T. (2009). Screening of Syphilis in the Subsaharan African blood donor :which strategy ? *Transfusion Clinique et Biologique.* doi:10.1016/j.tracli.2009.07.004

Tagny, C.T.; Owusu-ofori, S.; Mbanya, D. & Deneys, V. (2010). The blood donor in sub-Saharan Africa: a review. *Transf Med.* Vol.20, N°1, pp.1-10.

Tapko, S.B.; Sam, O. & Diarra-Nama ,A. (2005). Report on the status of blood safety in the WHO African region for 2004. Johannesburg: WHO Regional Office Africa.

Vall-Mayans, M.; Casals, M.; Vives, A.; Loureiro, E.; Armengol, P. & Sanz, B.(2006). Re-emergence of infectious syphilis among homosexual men and HIV co infection in Barcelona, 2002–2003. *Med Clin (Barc)* Vol.126, pp. 94–96.

Wendel, S.(1994). Current concepts on transmission of bacteria and parasites by blood components. *Vox Sang.* Vol.67 Suppl N°3, pp. 161–174.

WHO Department of HIV/AIDS. Geneva, Switzerland: WHO (2001). Global prevalence and incidence of selected curable sexually transmitted infections: overview and estimates. Available from: http://www.who.int/docstore/hiv/GRSTI/005.htm.

Workowski, K. A. & Berman, S.M. (2006). Sexually transmitted diseases treatment guidelines. *MMWR Recommend. Rep.* 55(RR-11), pp. 1-94.

World Health Organization. (2001). Global prevalence and incidence of selected curable sexually transmitted infections: overview and estimates. World Health Organization Geneva, Switzerland.
http://www.who.int/hiv/pub/sti/en/who_hiv_aids_2001.02.pdf.

World Health Organization (2006). The use of rapid syphilis tests. Geneva: the sexually transmitted diseases diagnostics initiative (SDI) by UNICEF/UNDP/World Bank/WHO (TDR/SDI/06.1. WHO/TDR)

Young, H. (2000). Guidelines for serological testing for syphilis. *Sex Transm Infect.,*Vol.76, pp.403-405.